T0357160

Praise for
Postdiabetic

"In all my years of writing and reading self-help books, it's not every day I get to talk about one as life-changing as what Eric and Rubén have put together. They've hit the nail on the head: it's not just a health-care mess we've got on our hands—it's a full-blown self-care meltdown. And diabetes? It's right there at the front, costing us dearly in so many ways. If you're pacing the floor over prediabetes or type 2 diabetes, or if it's keeping you up at night for someone you care about, this book is your new best friend. Dive in, and let's turn that worry into action."

— **Jack Canfield**, co-creator of the *New York Times* #1 best-selling series *Chicken Soup for the Soul*®

"One of the most powerful ways to enhance your brain is by improving your metabolism and your relationship with sugar. With 1 in 3 Americans being prediabetic, the significance of *Postdiabetic* by Eric Edmeades and Dr. Rubén Ruiz is profound. Dive into this book to elevate your overall health, brain function, and long-term cognitive well-being."

— **Jim Kwik**, *New York Times* best-selling author of *Limitless*

"As a passionate advocate for personal transformation, I am deeply impressed by *Postdiabetic* by Eric Edmeades and Dr. Rubén Ruiz. This book not only offers groundbreaking insights into reversing pre- and type 2 diabetes, but also empowers readers to make lasting changes in their relationship with health and nutrition. A must-read for anyone on a journey toward physical and emotional wellness."

— **Shelly Lefkoe**, co-founder of the Lefkoe Institute and co-author of *Hitting the Wall*

"*Postdiabetic* by Eric Edmeades and Dr. Rubén Ruiz is an essential guide for anyone looking to navigate the complexities of pre- and type 2 diabetes with a holistic approach. This book reflects a profound understanding of how diet impacts our overall health—a message I deeply resonate with in my own teachings and experiences."

— **Peggy Cappy**, creator of the PBS *Yoga for the Rest of Us* DVD series and the founder of Gentle Stretch Yoga

Postdiabetic

Postdiabetic

AN EASY-TO-FOLLOW
9-WEEK GUIDE TO
Reversing Prediabetes and Type 2 Diabetes

ERIC EDMEADES
AND RUBÉN RUIZ, M.D.

HAY HOUSE LLC
Carlsbad, California • New York City
London • Sydney • New Delhi

Copyright © 2024 by Catalystix, Ltd.

Published in the United States by: Hay House LLC, www.hayhouse.com® • P.O. Box 5100, Carlsbad, CA, 92018-5100

Project editor: Sally Mason-Swaab • *Indexer:* J S Editorial, LLC
*Cover design: the*Book Designers • *Interior design:* Karim J. Garcia
Scribe: Hal Clifford • *Publishing Manager*: Kacy Wren

Cataloging-in-Publication Data is on file at the Library of Congress.

Tradepaper ISBN: 978-1-4019-8030-6
E-book ISBN: 978-1-4019-7593-7
Audiobook ISBN: 978-1-4019-7594-4

10 9 8 7 6 5 4 3 2 1
1st edition, March 2024
2nd edition, March 2025

Printed in the United States of America

This product uses responsibly sourced papers and/or recycled materials. For more information, see www.hayhouse.com.

The authorized representative in the EU for product safety and compliance is Penguin Random House Ireland, Morrison Chambers, 32 Nassau Street, Dublin D02 YH68, Ireland. https://eu-contact.penguin.ie

This book is dedicated to all the frontline doctors, nurses, and support staff that have been working tirelessly and putting themselves at risk to keep us all safe during these difficult times.

Contents

PART III: SUSTAINING YOUR POSTDIABETIC JOURNEY

If you are a doctor or medical professional and would like to support your patients in their journey to postdiabetes, please contact us. Our programs make it easy for clients to make the lasting lifestyle changes required to reverse pre- and type 2 diabetes. If you would like to find out more, please visit **www.PostDiabetes.com/RX**.

Simply use your phone camera to scan this code to automatically visit the page.

Foreword

Recently Eric interviewed me for his WILDFIT members, and, after the interview, we discussed cases of reversal of type 2 diabetes. Eric pointed out that patients who normalize their blood sugar and stop all medication are still referred to as prediabetic. Instead, he suggested, we should refer to them as "*post*diabetic."

It was a light-bulb moment. They are clearly at risk for progression back to diabetes if they revert to their high-starch and high-sugar diets. Prediabetes is a well-defined state of blood sugar imbalance that includes glucose over 100, an increased waist size, high blood pressure, high triglycerides, and low HDL or good cholesterol.

As someone reverses their type 2 diabetes, they may, for a time, have measurements that fall into the prediabetic range, but they are *trending* in the other direction. This is an important distinction and should have a material impact upon any medical advice, intervention, or prescriptions they receive.

While the measurements on a particular day might be very similar for people dealing with pre- or postdiabetes, their trajectories are very different, and therefore, so should their medical advice be.

No book, on its own, is going to cure you of anything. This book is important and makes a number of compelling arguments, including that *type 2 diabetes is reversible* and that *postdiabetes should be treated differently from prediabetes*. In fact, I particularly like Eric and Rubén's argument that diabetes should be treated more like "an injury that can be *healed* than a chronic disease that must be *treated*."

Diabetes will, left unchecked, affect half of the people you know and is costing the economy hundreds of billions of dollars. The numbers are staggering and getting worse. In the 1970s, type 2 diabetes was virtually unknown for people under 40. Today, it has exploded to the point where half of the population will face type 2 diabetes, including 1 in 4 children.

In America, one out of every three dollars spent by Medicare is spent on diabetes, making it one of the most significant causes of the national debt.

Around the world, societies debate how to pay for healthcare or whether to have universal healthcare. A U.S. study predicted that the Patient Protection and Affordable Care Act (Obamacare) would save the American government $109 billion between 2012 and 2022. That sounds like a big number—$109 *billion* over ten years or around $10 billion per year—until you realize that diabetes and prediabetes cost Americans *$322 billion in 2012.*

Seventy-eight billion of that was lost productivity. The remaining $244 billion was for "excess medical costs"—that is, costs not otherwise incurred if people didn't have diabetes or prediabetes in the first place.

Big numbers are hard to digest. Here's another way to view that $322 billion: on average, diabetes costs every single American about a thousand dollars a year. Even worse, between 2007 and 2012, the cost of diabetes in America rose 48 percent.

And while we are talking about the personal cost of diabetes, there is another issue. As Rubén points out in this book, many people have no idea what diabetes really means. They receive the diagnosis and simply accept it as a life sentence and wonder which medications they will require.

A lifelong relationship with medication—whether pills or injections—is the smallest tip of the consequence iceberg when it comes to type 2 diabetes. If you, or anyone you know, are currently living with type 2 diabetes or prediabetes, it is incredibly important to know what that *means.*

Perhaps you know that pre- and type 2 diabetes means that your body is no longer processing sugar efficiently or effectively, either because your body is resisting insulin or not producing enough. On the surface, this seems fairly innocuous; surely there is a medication that can sort this out. Medication can help reduce blood sugar and future complications such as nerve damage, kidney damage, heart and blood vessel disease, Alzheimer's, eye damage, and early death, but it does not eliminate them. The only thing that can do that is to reverse type 2 diabetes with food and exercise.

If you are concerned about or are living with type 2 diabetes, please buy another copy of this book and give it to your doctor. Type 2 diabetes should no longer be seen as a *chronic disease* but, rather, *an injury* from which you can recover.

Dr. Ruiz and Eric have done an excellent job making this argument, and they have provided an effective step-by-step program for becoming *post*diabetic.

Don't just read this book. Read it, follow the steps, and then pass it on to someone else who needs to know.

— **Mark Hyman, M.D.**
Head of Strategy and Innovation
Cleveland Clinic Center for Functional Medicine
New York Times best-selling author of
Food: What the Heck Should I Eat?

Introduction

Introducing Rubén Ruiz, M.D.

Early one afternoon in 2015, I pulled onto the I-10 freeway in Los Angeles. Man, was I tired. I tucked my second Starbucks grande coffee of the day into the car's cup holder. I felt tired a lot back then. I was sleepy all the time, drinking coffee like crazy just to stay alert.

Those days I never felt that great but figured that's just what getting older meant. Over the years, the needle on the scale had crept up from 160 pounds to 250. Gaining 90 pounds didn't happen overnight. It was imperceptible from day to day.

Other things about my health were slipping too. I had high blood pressure, another problem that had slowly crept up on me. I had developed sleep apnea and didn't sleep well. My cholesterol, triglycerides, and hemoglobin A1C blood sugar measurements were all up.

In the course of a decade, my health had deteriorated to the point that I was on 10 medications, apparently forever.* I had signed up to be a healer, and I couldn't even heal myself.

---

* Here's the list of medications Rubén was taking:
Metformin 500mg twice daily for diabetes
Triamterene and hydrochlorothiazide (Maxzide) 75mg/50mg daily for severe hypertension and early heart failure
Carvedilol (Coreg) 25mg twice daily for severe hypertension, early heart failure, and palpitations
Atorvastatin (Lipitor) 40mg daily for dyslipidemia (elevated triglycerides and cholesterol)
Omeprazole (Prilosec) 40mg daily for chronic acid reflux
Tamsulosin (Flomax) 0.4mg daily for benign prostatic hypertrophy
Levothyroxine sodium (Synthroid) 100mcg daily for hypothyroidism
Fluticasone propionate nasal (Flonase) two actuations to each nostril daily for chronic allergies
Loratadine (Claritin) 1 daily for chronic allergies
Zolpidem (Ambien) 10mg at bedtime for insomnia

I wasn't happy about the weight gain but hadn't been able to control it. I'd tried many diets, but they didn't seem to work. Was being tired related to being overweight? Maybe. I'm a doctor, but I honestly didn't know. Nothing in medical school had taught me about any potential connection.

The traffic on the I-10 was thick, but it moved steadily along. It was hard to focus. I was just so tired . . .

There was a terrible noise. I had fallen asleep at the wheel and drifted into the HOV lane. I had hit a motorcyclist.

I leaped from the car. "I'm so sorry. I'm so sorry!" I said again and again. To this day I thank God that the driver was traveling slow enough that the result wasn't catastrophic. The motorcyclist was shaken, and both the car and the bike were damaged. I couldn't apologize enough. I felt awful. He and I both had been lucky.

A week later, my own car was still at the body shop. Now behind the wheel of a rented Audi, I pulled onto the I-10 as usual, and headed north with a 20-ounce Starbucks coffee beside me. As usual, I was tired. So tired.

This time when I fell asleep, the car drifted right, hitting an SUV and totaling it. Somehow, the driver was all right. So was I.

Or was I? Two accidents in a week? What was going on?

Shortly after those two automobile accidents, I, Dr. Rubén Ruiz, met my co-author, Eric Edmeades. I was curious about Eric's work, and I joined his program.

Eric was surprised to hear that I, a medical doctor, wanted to learn about his nutrition-based approach to health and wellness. The truth is, nutrition isn't taught in medical schools unless a student happens to take some elective classes. It's a huge blind spot for doctors, including me.

As I worked through Eric's program and found success in it, I realized that I was no longer tired all the time. I soon found that I no longer felt sluggish waking up in the morning and didn't feel like I needed a nap in the afternoon. Within 90 days I was sleeping better, my blood sugars were dropping, and soon I was off all but one of my medications. I lost weight, gained energy, and felt so much better.

That is when it hit me: diabetes had been making me tired. I had been diabetic for 10 years, and type 2 diabetes was why I nearly killed two innocent bystanders, and myself, on the freeway.

Being sick, being overweight, and having low energy was not only inconvenient; it was dangerous. And it was embarrassing, because I am a doctor.

Together, Eric and I changed my life. It had been on a course of slow medical deterioration for a decade. Most importantly, we reversed the course of the type 2 diabetes that slowly had been ravaging me. I finally grasped what the phrase "physician, heal thyself" meant. Because that was what I had done.

And now, for the first time since I was fresh out of medical school, I really felt like I could help people—people with diabetes. I was reborn as a doctor with a new sense of mission. I could help them get better. I could help them feel better. And I could help them reduce or get rid of all the side-effect-causing medication that I used to prescribe.

Introducing Eric Edmeades, Founder, WILDFIT

As I learned more about Rubén's story and saw his success in rolling back diabetes, I realized I'd heard this before. Multiple times. My program has helped thousands of people, some of whom had type 2 diabetes. Many people, after participating in our programs, reported that they had visited their doctors and been told they were no longer diabetic; their symptoms had improved to the degree that they were "prediabetic."

This terminology struck me as logically flawed. After all, if you had previously been diabetic, you couldn't regress to being prediabetic. No, what our clients had done is move through diabetes to something else. They were on the other side of diabetes. They were trending in the other direction.

They were what we now call *"post*diabetic."

Postdiabetic is a term that does not exist in the medical literature—not yet. But it's a reality that we—Eric and Rubén—have seen happen again and again.

And it is not a simple matter of semantics. A postdiabetic patient might have measurements that fall in the prediabetic range, but they are trending in the other direction, and this should influence any medical advice or medication they receive.

Once we realized we were looking at a new, or at least unrecognized, medical phenomenon, we felt we had to do more. We knew we possessed a critical counter-message to the conventional narrative around diabetes, and we were determined to share it: *you can reverse your type 2 diabetes* or, as we like to say, *#postdiabeticispossible*.

One of the most compelling observations that led us to write this book is the way we hear commentary about how people are "struck down" by disease. People say someone was "struck down" by cancer or heart disease or diabetes, and that seemed wrong to us. Now, if you are attacked by Ebola, or COVID-19, or even the flu virus, it's fair to say you were not at fault. You were literally attacked by a disease—struck down. (It is interesting to note, with this example, that early evidence coming from the COVID-19 pandemic suggests that the virus is much more dangerous for those with compromised health or immune systems, particularly those with diabetes and/or obesity.)

On the other hand, heart disease, diabetes, and even cancer are sometimes called lifestyle diseases—they are afflictions we bring upon ourselves, in many cases, by the choices we make. When we see individuals who appear to have made bad choices, it's easy to judge them. Have you ever winced when an overweight person sits next to you on an airplane and thought, *Why do they do that to themselves?*

But as I worked with more and more people on changing their relationship with food, I learned that this judgment is way off the mark. While people are free to make their own food and exercise choices, it has become crystal clear that the food industry has been doing everything they can to boost their profits without a second thought to the impact on individual health or the social costs. The food industry, as we will discuss further in this book, is just as manipulative and unethical as the tobacco industry ever was, maybe even more so.

Even the term *lifestyle disease* is an attempt to shift the blame from a profit-motivated food industry onto the consumer.

If you are, as you read this book, suffering with a "lifestyle" disease such as type 2 diabetes, obesity, hypertension, or even many autoimmune diseases, we would like to tell you two important things:

1.   It is *NOT* your fault.

2.   It *IS* your responsibility to turn things around now.

The truth is that the responsibility for the pain, discomfort, suffering, and economic devastation caused by type 2 diabetes lies squarely at the feet of food manufacturers and their lobbyists. In this book we will show you how you can take responsibility for your own quality of life and defend yourself from these bad actors.

Who Are We and Why Did We Write This Book?

This book is premised on our belief that type 2 diabetes should not be considered a chronic disease that requires lifelong treatment and medication but that, instead, it should be viewed as a repetitive stress injury that *can be healed*.

When we see people suffering with type 2 diabetes—having to take medication, carefully watch exactly what they eat, and inject themselves daily—we don't simply see the pain in the present. We see the painful and difficult future ahead of them.

Today, medical professionals and their patients regard type 2 diabetes as a life sentence, and for many, it is. People with diabetes do not just face current health problems. They face a future plagued by eyesight challenges, circulatory issues, potential amputations, heart disease, and a slew of other, associated health problems.*†

---

* According to the Mayo Clinic, there are a number of factors that increase your risk of diabetes. Being overweight is a main risk factor for type 2 diabetes, but there are other factors:
Fat distribution. If you store fat mainly in the abdomen, you have a greater risk of type 2 diabetes than if you store fat elsewhere, such as in your hips and thighs. Your risk of type 2 diabetes rises if you're a man with a waist circumference above 40 inches (101.6 centimeters) or a woman with a waist that's greater than 35 inches (88.9 centimeters).
Inactivity. The less active you are, the greater your risk of type 2 diabetes. Physical activity helps you control your weight, uses up glucose as energy, and makes your cells more sensitive to insulin.
Family history. The risk of type 2 diabetes increases if your parent or sibling has type 2 diabetes.
Race. Although it's unclear why, people of certain races—including Black, Hispanic, American Indian, and Asian American people—are more likely to develop type 2 diabetes than white people are.
Age. The risk of type 2 diabetes increases as you get older, especially after age 45. That's probably because people tend to exercise less, lose muscle mass, and gain weight as they age. But type 2 diabetes is also increasing dramatically among children, adolescents, and younger adults.
Prediabetes. Prediabetes is a condition in which your blood sugar level is higher than normal but not high enough to be classified as diabetes. Left untreated, prediabetes often progresses to type 2 diabetes.
Gestational diabetes. If you developed gestational diabetes when you were pregnant, your risk of developing type 2 diabetes increases. If you gave birth to a baby weighing more than 9 pounds (4 kilograms), you're also at risk of type 2 diabetes.
Polycystic ovary syndrome. For women, having polycystic ovary syndrome—a common condition characterized by irregular menstrual periods, excess hair growth, and obesity—increases the risk of diabetes.

† Diabetes causes many conditions, including microvascular complications such as retinopathy (blindness), nephropathy (renal failure and dialysis), neuropathy (nerve failure, numbness, and amputations), and macrovascular complications: coronary vascular disease, myocardial infarction (heart attack), cerebrovascular disease, stroke, Alzheimer's disease, and death.

We see this, and we feel like screaming, *No, this is not a life sentence!* It's merely a statement of how things are now. We want to change the way people see type 2 diabetes so they see it as an injury that you can recover from rather than a chronic disease that must be "managed" for life.

Who are we to say this? We've come from different directions that intersect at this conclusion. Rubén has been a medical internist for 37 years and an assistant professor of medicine at the University of California, Los Angeles before going into private practice. He served as chief medical officer for a series of clinics in Los Angeles before starting his own, which principally serves Medicare and Medicaid patients, along with the uninsured.

Rubén met Eric through one of Eric's health coaching programs. Eric was born into a medical family in South Africa and immigrated as a child to Canada, where he received his education. Eric is an entrepreneur and has owned businesses in mobile computing, Hollywood film production, military research and development, and high-fidelity medical simulation before founding WILDFIT, a health coaching and transformation company. Through WILDFIT, Eric has helped (as of this writing) more than 50,000 people in 130 countries transform their health by changing their relationship with food. In 2018, the Canadian Senate presented Eric with a Senate 150 Medal in recognition of his work to improve the quality of people's lives around the world.

Both of us struggled with food-related issues earlier in our lives. In 1991, Eric was his own first client: overweight, suffering, in pain, on multiple medications, and staring down the barrel of a prescribed surgery. Luckily, he happened to have a very powerful conversation with a couple of friends about food. Thirty days later he'd lost 30 pounds, all his symptoms were gone, and he no longer required surgery. This experience inspired a deep curiosity. How was it, he thought, that he had spent almost a decade visiting doctors and specialists who prescribed a variety of ineffective medications but offered no advice about food?

Rubén, whose story we told you at the beginning of this Introduction, did not think he could reverse his diabetes at all, but

then he did just that by working with Eric and changing his relationship with food. Today, both of us see the positive effects of the
changes we describe in this book manifesting in Rubén's patients
and in Eric's clients alike.

And yet, in his Los Angeles clinic, Rubén has seen a disheartening change in the way people respond to a diagnosis of diabetes.
It used to be that people were afraid, just as they would be afraid of
a cancer diagnosis. But now diabetes is so common, so prevalent—
at least a third[1] of all Americans are diabetic or prediabetic—that
patients don't think much about it. They just figure they'll have
to take a pill for the rest of their lives. They don't understand how
devastating diabetes can be for them and their families, and they
don't understand that this diagnosis—this "fate"—is something
they can change.

+ + +

*Eric: When we first started working with people on their
food psychology, we saw many positive results that we expected
to see as people developed a healthier relationship with food:
weight loss, better energy, improved fertility, and improved
cognition.*

*But every now and then, something monumental would
happen.*

*I remember getting a letter from a client who said that their
doctor had taken them off their blood pressure medication.
Another day I received one from a client who had been living
with arthritic pain for 20 years, and it had simply vanished.
There was a client who said the allergies she had suffered from
her whole life were now gone.*

*We received so many messages like this, messages describ-
ing extraordinary results, that after a while they didn't feel
all that extraordinary. I remember receiving another remarkable health turnaround letter and not being all that surprised.
I thought, Oh, look, another letter with diabetes reversal,
and then I caught myself and realized how incredibly special*

it was to receive these letters and how important our message had become.

The one report that kept showing up again and again was from people who had been diagnosed as type 2 diabetics who were no longer type 2 but were now being labeled "prediabetic."

That just struck me wrong. Prediabetes means you are "trending toward diabetes." But these people were trending away from diabetes. I explained this to one of our clients who was in this situation. "Your numbers might indicate you're in a range that could be considered prediabetic," I said, "but you are not prediabetic. You are trending in the other direction. Therefore you are postdiabetic."

"That's it!" he said. "I am going to go tell my doctor I'm postdiabetic!"

From that point on, we began explaining to our previously type 2 diabetes clients that perhaps they were postdiabetic. By giving the condition a name, we were also making it real and achievable. This wasn't theory; we were seeing it every day, and that evidence set us on the course to writing this book. Further, the medical advice a doctor might give someone who is prediabetic (trending toward full-blown type 2 diabetes) might be very different from the advice they might give to someone with the same numbers but trending away from diabetes.

Today, when a patient walks into the clinic and tells Rubén that he doesn't sleep well, he snores all the time, he's short of breath when he goes up the stairs, and he's a little overweight, Rubén feels deeply for them. Because he was there! That's who he was, and over a decade his diabetes crept up on him. But he knows now it doesn't have to be that way. Many of his patients don't even know what diabetes is. And when Rubén tells them that they can take a different path, that they can heal themselves, their eyes light up.

Eric, for his part, was struggling with how to help even more people. To wake up to yet more messages from people who had turned their diabetes around, yet walk down the street and see people who likely were or would soon be diagnosed with type 2 diabetes was incredibly frustrating. This book is meant to close the gap, to help those people who might otherwise have lived with type 2 diabetes—and the related consequences—for the rest of their lives.

If you're reading this book, you or someone you care about likely already has received a diagnosis of being diabetic or prediabetic. You're probably worried about that, and with good reason. In this book we're going to reframe the way you think about diabetes. As we've said, we are suggesting that you treat it like an injury, not a chronic disease, which means it is something you can recover from.

You might wonder why, if type 2 diabetes is reversible, it is commonly treated as a lifelong condition, and the answer might shock you: It is being treated that way because it is incredibly profitable to treat it that way. It is a lot more profitable to sell drugs to treat lifelong conditions than to show people how to turn them around.

Things don't have to be like this.

To prove the point, we're going to show you documented case studies that demonstrate this condition is recoverable.

And then, having made the point that *post*diabetes is possible, we will give you a solid step-by-step plan that just might reverse the condition for you. The process is simple and straightforward, and it will guide you through some manageable lifestyle changes that will give your body the opportunity to heal.

Everything that you need to recover from your diagnosis is in this book *except* your determination to stick with the program. We will make it as easy as possible; we won't ask you to make sweeping changes all at once, count calories, weigh your food, or undertake strenuous workouts. We will be working on powerful, proven, effective, and incremental steps that will help you get immediate results and long-lasting transformation.

We will also talk about willpower. Willpower is not a long-term strategy. Willpower can start things off and simulate change, but to create lasting results, we have to go much deeper than willpower. If, at any stage of this book, you feel like you don't have the willpower to move forward or to stop eating a particular food, please watch this video by Eric.‡

This book is not a miracle between two covers. You will not read the book and be magically cured. It is a practical, step-by-step process for improving your health and reversing type 2 diabetes without supplements, drugs, or heavy exercise.

We also want to end the shame around diabetes and obesity. If you are struggling with your weight and or diabetes, we have an important message for you: *it is not your fault.*

Large profit-seeking corporations—soft drink manufacturers, sugar growers, and pharmaceutical companies—make billions at the expense of our health. You will learn exactly what they are up to and how you can combat them and regain your own health while improving conditions for generations to come.

As Dr. Mark Hyman wrote in the Foreword, diabetes is catastrophically expensive. It cost Americans $322 billion in 2012 alone, almost three times all the savings Patient Protection and Affordable Care Act was predicted to accumulate over a decade. Three-quarters of that cost was medical expenditures. Numbers that big are hard to digest, so look at it this way: diabetes costs every American, even those *without* diabetes, $1,000 every year via funding from unemployment taxes, reduced productivity, and increased absenteeism. And the cost is rising steadily.

One could quibble with these numbers, at least around the edges. You could say our population is growing and aging, and diabetes tends to affect older people, so that might explain some of this rise. But you cannot argue with the simple massiveness of this problem. So think—just from a dollars-and-cents perspective—about what a difference it will make to healthcare systems and worldwide economies if we can collectively bend that growth trend, and even reverse it, by changing the way we understand diabetes, the way we think about it, and the way we treat it.

---

‡   If you are struggling with willpower, please check out this video from Eric about food psychology and how to easily and permanently change your relationship with food: www.postdiabetes.com/resources/willpower.

How to Get the Most out of This Book

In the pages to come, we make the case that type 2 diabetes is something that an irresponsible food and beverage manufacturing industry does to people; it is not self-inflicted. Then we show you why what has been done to you is not permanent, even though the medical establishment treats it that way. We will include case studies from people from all walks of life who have overcome type 2 diabetes, so you will know in your heart that you, too, can recover. Finally, we give you a step-by-step process for turning things around over the next nine weeks.

To get the most out of this book, read it in order and keep the following things in mind.

First, plan to teach what you learn. Memory works in a funny way. When you read something with the intention of teaching it to someone else, you store it more permanently in your memory. If you know in your mind and your heart with whom you might want to share this information, you will learn it more holistically. Decide now with whom you want to share it. Sure, we'd love for you to buy more copies of this book and give them away. But we'd also love for you to simply teach others what you have learned yourself.

Second, we recommend that you use a journal along with the book. Even if you write in it only once a week, log the experience. This could mean writing in your own private journal; it could mean documenting on Instagram or Facebook. What matters is that you create a record of your history. You begin by saying, "Today is the day I decide to turn my situation around," and then each week you write a little bit about your experience. (If you decide to blog or post your journey on social media, please use the hashtag #postdiabeticispossible so that we can find your story and see how you are doing.)

Third, celebrate progress. Progress is fundamental to human motivation and inspiration: To get the most out of this program, you must recognize progress wherever it shows up. We know that your ultimate goal is to become *post*diabetic, to get so far from diabetes that a doctor couldn't even say your symptoms are pre-diabetic. But there are a bunch of other outcomes that are also positive and that we want you to recognize if they happen to you.

For example:

- What if you suddenly found yourself with more energy?

- What if you found yourself falling asleep more easily at bedtime?

- What if you fell asleep when you wanted to and stayed sharp and awake when you wanted?

- What if you woke up feeling recharged?

- What if your circulation improved?

- What if the aches and pains in your joints faded away?

- What if your inflammation disappeared?

- What if you were able to reduce or even eliminate your medications?*

- What if you were exposed to a coronavirus and your body's immune system fought it effectively so that you had no or very few symptoms?

Each of these things are small steps of progress on the way to your ultimate goal. If you can begin noticing that progress—both the mental progress you make and how your body is working—it will lead to increased motivation and better willpower.

That's important, because there may come a time when you want to eat something you know you really shouldn't. If you have no sense of the progress you've made, it will be easier to give in at that moment. On the other hand, if you have a very clear catalog

---

* Please only make changes to your medication with medical supervision.

of the progress you've made the entire way, you're far more likely to stick to the program.

Fourth, get absolutely clear on your "why." For some people the why is personal. They don't want to be in pain anymore. They don't want to take multiple dangerous oral medications or insulin injections anymore. They don't want to fight with themselves about food anymore. For other people it's more social. They want to be there for their children and their grandchildren. Knowing your why, your motivation, gives you the energy you need to do this work.

Fifth, don't read ahead. In Part II we give you week-by-week instructions. At the end of each chapter in Part II, we ask you *not to read ahead* until you have completed that week. In that part of the book, you should only read one chapter per week. We do this for a very specific reason: We understand what works. We don't want you to concern yourself with what you *will* have to do in the future. We only want you to focus on what you *do* have to do *now* and to see the results that come from that. Those incremental successes prepare you for each week to follow.

Get help. Don't do this alone. Please join our online community at **www.postdiabetes.com/facebook** or, if you could use a little extra support, book yourself a session with a registered facilitator or certified doctors at **www.postdiabetes.com/findafacilitator**.

Do these things, and three months from now you'll be healthier than you ever thought possible.

PART I

IT'S NOT YOUR FAULT

CHAPTER 1

How Did This Happen to You?

Your diabetes is not your fault.

Before we explain why, let's take a short detour into what type 2 diabetes is.

The *Oxford English Dictionary* defines diabetes as "a disease in which the body's ability to produce or respond to the hormone insulin is impaired, resulting in abnormal metabolism of carbohydrates and elevated levels of glucose in the blood and urine." This definition is why many people, including doctors, are not clear about what diabetes *actually* is.

Let's put it in layperson's terms.

Type 2 diabetes is considered a chronic disease wherein the body does not use insulin well. The primary causes of type 2 diabetes are diet and lifestyle. Formally referred to as "adult-onset diabetes," type 2 diabetes is at epidemic levels in young people too as a result of recent changes in lifestyle and diet habits around the world. (Type 1 diabetes, previously known as "juvenile" or "insulin-dependent" diabetes has different causes and does not appear to be reversible.)

We believe that type 2 diabetes is reversible in the vast majority of cases. While those with type 1 diabetes cannot, to our knowledge, become postdiabetic in the way that those with type

2 can, we believe that the strategies included in this book can also help those with type 1 by improving their overall health and reducing their dependence upon insulin injections.

Understanding type 2 diabetes begins with understanding how we use sugar as a fuel. We have three fuel sources: sugar, fat, and protein, all of which can be converted to sugar and then transported by the blood. When we take in sugar, our body seeks to use it as efficiently and quickly as possible. When we take in too much too often, the body can suffer what we, the authors, think of as a repetitive stress injury, resulting in type 2 diabetes.

Diabetes begins at the cellular level. A cell needs an ocean to live in. It needs access to food, access to oxygen, and to be able to get rid of waste. The beauty of the body is it provides this ocean through the circulatory system: the arteries and veins and capillaries that provide an ocean to every cell.

In the simplest terms, type 2 diabetes is a problem of elevated blood sugar that can lead to insulin sensitivity issues. Insulin, a hormone made by the pancreas, opens doors or pathways for glucose to get into cells. The cells decide if they are in need of fuel or are already topped up. If topped up, the insulin induces the fat storage mechanism in the cells. In time, the fat in the cells mucks up the mechanics of glucose entry. The fat guy is in the doorway, and glucose can't get in.

Since the glucose can't get in, it stays outside in the blood, making the blood sticky. This is the first of three problems that are caused by elevated blood sugar. Hormones and other things that travel around in the blood get stuck to each other and are not available to cells. Sticky blood, nonfunctional insulin, and a fat guy in the doorway combine to create insulin insensitivity.

Second, because the blood is sticky, it clogs up capillaries, so the blood can't get to certain places in the body. If they don't have good blood flow, cells are going to die.

Third, all that sugar brings water with it. If we've got a lot of sugar in the cells and the matrix around the cells, that causes swelling. It's like what happens in a traffic jam on a freeway—nobody can move.

These three effects of high blood sugar start the whole process of damage. The cells start saying, "I've got no food, I can't get rid of my waste, and I'm going to die." Nerves start dying off slowly, eyes start deteriorating, and kidneys start failing.

While the effects of type 2 diabetes contribute to problems like cardiovascular disease, the potential development of cancer, and circulatory problems, what's become even more obvious is that type 2 diabetes affects our immune system, as shown by how susceptible diabetics are in the world of COVID-19.

Even before COVID-19, the effects of diabetes were a problem. Diabetics are very prone to infections. A diabetic's immune system doesn't work well because cells don't get enough energy from glucose to function well. Blood proteins don't function well because of this stickiness. Swelling caused by excess sugar in the blood further restricts circulation, making everything worse.

+ + +

Before sugar became widely available, humans only had occasional exposure to it, mostly through seasonal fruits, root vegetables, and wild honey. Our hormones evolved to deal with the energy systems in our body, including insulin and glucagon, both produced by the pancreas.

Insulin is produced when we consume sugars (carbohydrates), and glucagon is produced when we are running low on sugar so that we can switch to fat metabolism.

Traditionally, glucagon used to do the lion's share of the work; our ancestors spent the majority of any year producing glucagon and only produced insulin on the rare occasions that carbohydrate-rich foods (fruit, root vegetables, honey) were in season and consumed.

Today, we have more than inverted that ratio so that most people spend their entire year producing insulin to process all the sugars (sugar, fruit, bread, pasta, and other carbohydrate foods) that we eat in the modern diet. Far from spending most of our time producing glucagon, many people rarely if ever produce glucagon. This is a serious problem.

Our bodies evolved complex systems designed to increase our odds of survival. Our ancestors lived in very difficult and dangerous times with a multitude of threats to their survival, including food supply issues and harsh environmental conditions.

Most of our evolution took place in sub-Saharan Africa. Starvation was a regular threat that was particularly serious during the winter season when there was a lack of rain and, correspondingly, a reduction in the food supply.

Homo sapiens adapted to survive these cyclical weather patterns—seasons—and as a result, we have dual-function organs like the pancreas. The pancreas changes behavior depending on which season we are in, and it determines that primarily by the foods we are eating.

If one of your ancestors found themselves eating large quantities of fruit, their body would deduce that the season was autumn and that the pancreas should primarily be focused on producing insulin to break down the carbohydrates that are so plentiful at that time of year.

This worked out very well for our ancestors because our bodies would, when we ate more sugar than was needed or usable on a particular day, store those calories for use in the future as glycogen, in the muscles for the medium term and as fat for the long term.

This adaptation made it possible for our ancestors to survive the drought-heavy winter months by storing energy and water (fat). This meant that they would not be dependent on the daily consumption of food or water and increased their odds of survival and, therefore, the passing on of their genes.

And then, when the fruits and carbohydrates disappeared as quickly as they had arrived, our ancestors' bodies changed gears; their pancreases switched to the winter season and started producing glucagon, putting their bodies into ketosis (fat burning).

Because it is an absence of sugar that causes the change, switching to glucagon production is not as quick as the switch from glucagon to insulin production. Should one of our ancestors have stumbled upon a beehive in midwinter and gorged on the hive honey, the pancreas would switch gears immediately to produce the insulin needed to process the honey. It may then take some time for the pancreas to slow down and stop insulin production and resume production of glucagon. During this lag period, we often experience powerful sugar cravings; this appears to be an attempt by the body to motivate more carb consumption to increase the odds of surviving through the winter.

This is an important distinction that will come up again when we discuss our plan for reversing type 2 diabetes, and it provides a vital clue to unlocking the mysteries surrounding weight loss.

This evolutionary development—the pancreas, an organ that produces two different hormones, glucagon and insulin, depending on what foods we consume—is really extraordinary. It is a wonder of human development that we came up with such an elegant solution, rather than, say, developing separate organs to do these two very different jobs.

Further, the pancreas supports both the digestive (producing digestive enzymes) and endocrine (regulating blood sugar) systems; it is a truly remarkable organ. Understanding the pancreas and its role in our ancestors' survival of seasons lies at the core of how we can reverse diabetes.

Diabetes can manifest a couple of ways. For instance, for some people the pancreas does not produce enough insulin. They eat a phenomenal amount of carbohydrate foods, and the pancreas just can't keep up. The other common situation is that the pancreas does, in fact, produce enough insulin, but it isn't having the effect it should.

As we have discussed, when you eat sugar in any form, your pancreas creates insulin, which allows sugar fuel to enter cells. We burn it like a car burns gasoline. Sugar is used wherever it's needed in the body—it's really fast energy. The problem comes when there is too much sugar. The body has to do something with it. It will store it as glycogen in the liver, and in the muscles, and in the organs, but eventually they fill up. It's as if you have a full tank of gas in your car while it's parked in the garage, and you're trying to put more gas into the tank. The body has to do something else with that fuel—sugar—so it converts it to fat.

The fat is stored everywhere, beginning in the pancreas and liver. It's stored microscopically throughout the body, so people begin to put on weight. Our bodies are very smart; we store fat first in places where it might be useful (protecting the abdomen) and then in places where it won't inhibit movement or flexibility (legs, bum, upper arms).

All this fat inhibits the ability of insulin to work, so the pancreas has to produce more and more insulin to handle the sugar that keeps coming in every time you eat. Like an alcoholic who needs to drink more and more to get the same effect, your body needs more and more insulin to process sugar. The body begins to become what we call *insulin resistant.*

At this point, the hemoglobin in the blood can become covered with sugar, which starts to cause all kinds of problems in your body, including circulatory problems that can lead to strokes, heart attacks, amputations, infections, peripheral nerve disease, and retinal eye disease.

Doctors use a test, called hemoglobin A1C, which measures how much sugar the blood is carrying. If the test comes in around 5 percent, that's okay. But if we start to see numbers around 7 percent or 9 percent, we know the insulin is not working well.* The sugar is gumming up the works and slowing down your body and blood flow. And then things stop working. Your body's defenses don't work properly. Your organs lose efficiency. The conventional treatment is to give people insulin injections or metformin, which is an approach that treats the symptoms, rather than the cause. In a sense, living out of balance by consuming too much carbohydrate-rich food too regularly might strain the pancreas and other related systems. This is why we suggest that diabetes is rather more like a repetitive stress injury than a disease.

The pancreas didn't evolve for extended and continuous consumption of carbohydrates. It gets tired. It is forced to overproduce.

---

* The most widely used clinical test to estimate blood glucose control is measurement of glycolated hemoglobin (also called A1C, hemoglobin A1C, glycohemoglobin or HbA1C). A1C reflects average blood glucose over the entire 120-day lifespan of the red blood cell, but it correlates best with average blood glucose over the previous 8 to 12 weeks. The A1C is the test that best predicts problems that occur as the result of having sugar caramelize the body. The higher the A1C, the more risk there is of developing problems. Normal is less than 5.7. Prediabetes, or the beginning of a rise in problem risk, occurs at an A1C of 5.7. Diabetes occurs with an A1C over 6.4, which means a marked rise in risk.

The insulin loses effectiveness, and the pancreas tries to produce even more insulin until, perhaps, it simply can't.

Remember how unnatural this situation is as you progress in this book. The pancreas should be producing glucagon most of the time and insulin only occasionally. The key to our successful approach to diabetes lies in supporting the pancreas to do the job it is meant to do rather than forcing it to adapt to abnormal conditions. We will come back to this in future chapters.

As you proceed through this book, please come back to these two ideas:

1. The pancreas is an outstanding organ and incredibly good at its jobs, as long as we ask it to do the right jobs at roughly the right ratio.

2. Asking the pancreas to do the wrong jobs strains or injures it and returning it to normal function just might allow it to heal and repair itself.

SHIFTING THE BLAME: ACT I

You may be old enough to remember what it was like to have sugar as a kid. It was a treat to get an ice-cream cone or some candy. Perhaps you have seen the now-viral video[†] of a toddler tasting ice cream for the first time. The video captures the intense feelings of joy and the powerful cravings that are stimulated by the near-radioactive levels of sweetness.

In the past, sugar was clearly associated with particular foods, usually dessert foods. Today, the food industry has at least 65 different terms[‡] for the various sugars that are introduced into all kinds of foods. Historically, Americans consumed about five pounds of sugar per person per year. Today, we consume more than 150 pounds of sugar per person per year. We're addicted to the stuff, and our bodies are not built to handle it in these quantities. Most damaging is that because we did evolve the ability to

---

† You can watch the video at www.PostDiabetes.com/videos/FirstIceCream

‡ To download a free copy of *The Hidden Names of Sugar*, please visit www.PostDiabetes.com/65Names

process sugar binges, the consequences of this overconsumption are not immediate enough to stop us in our tracks. And so we keep eating the stuff and allowing it to be added to our food, where it stimulates our appetite and makes us want to eat more.

In the 1950s, as we began to eat more sugar, there were some disturbing developments in the food and health sciences. Researchers began to become aware of the role that sugar plays in dental cavities. At the same time research began to suggest that, at a minimum, there was a correlation between sugar consumption and coronary heart disease and cholesterol buildup. In fact, there were strong suggestions that sugar might be to blame.

An organization called the Sugar Research Foundation began commissioning a variety of studies to, in essence, preserve the sugar industry's market share. Through the foundation, the industry sponsored research that distracted Americans away from the bad news about sugar—research that ostensibly cleared sugar from any relationship with coronary artery disease and that in turn suggested that fat and cholesterol were the bigger culprits. They published a paper saying just that in the *Journal of the American Medical Association*.

Publicly the sugar industry was saying, "Wow, we really want to dig into this research and help people have better lives." But behind the scenes, they were working to preserve market share, and in so doing they saw an opportunity to actually increase market share by taking advantage of the gap that would be caused if people cut back on fat. Their plan was to preserve their own market share by protecting the reputation of sugar and then score a bigger market share by damaging the reputation of fat. It was a cunning plan, and it really worked.

In 1954, the president of the Sugar Research Foundation, Henry Haas, gave a speech to the American Society of Sugar Beet Technologists describing a phenomenal opportunity:

> Leading nutritionists are pointing out the chemical connection between [Americans'] high-fat diet and the formation of cholesterol, which partly plugs our arteries and capillaries, restricts the flow of blood, and causes

high blood pressure and heart trouble . . . if you put [the middle-aged man] on a low-fat diet, it takes just five days for the blood cholesterol to get down to where it should be . . . If the carbohydrate industries were to recapture this 20 percent of the calories in the U.S. diet (the difference between the 40 percent which fat has and the 20 percent which it ought to have) and if sugar maintained its present share of the carbohydrate market, this change would mean an increase in the per capita consumption of sugar more than a third with a tremendous improvement in general health.[1]

But there was one thing that Haas left out: these "leading nutritionists" were in his pocket.

He predicted that if Americans cut fat consumption from the present (at that time) 40 percent of average calories consumed to 20 percent of calories, then sugar could step in and fill that 20 percent gap. That would result in a one-third increase in sugar consumption. It was a huge business opportunity.

For more than a decade, the industry continued to fund research designed to challenge any assertion that sugar caused heart disease. In one such example, as discussed in a 2016 *Time* magazine expose of the sugar industry, a Sugar Research Foundation–funded study prepared by two Harvard researchers attempted to shift the blame for heart disease from sugar to fat. They disingenuously argued that existing animal studies linking sugar to heart disease were limited, the data wasn't really up to snuff, and the real problem was fat.

Until 1982, the *New England Journal of Medicine* did not require funding disclosures for published papers or studies. And so, this research was published in a prestigious journal, became lore, and gave birth to the low-fat food industry while taking our eyes off the sugar industry and the harm it was causing.[2]

Stanton Glantz, one of the authors of the "study," told *The New York Times* that "it was a very smart thing the sugar industry did, because review papers, especially if you get them published in a very prominent journal, tend to shape the overall scientific discussion."

He was right. Americans came to believe fat, not sugar, caused increased cholesterol and heart disease. This was a brilliant move by the sugar industry. And it was not their last move.

WE EVOLVED TO CRAVE SUGAR

So why did the sugar industry do this to us?

Let's look at that question from the food company executives' point of view. If your product is threatened by cutting-edge science that verges on saying it is unhealthy if not downright dangerous, that's a problem. You have stakeholders to answer to. You've got an industry to support. You want to defend yourself, so what can you do? Well, you can potentially preserve your market share by commissioning reports and studies that take the eye off sugar and place the blame on fat.

As we have just discussed, this is just what sugar executives did in the 1960s.

But why stop there?

Understanding the human relationship with sugar, and how the body reacts to it, creates additional opportunities for improved profits.

Why do we like sugar or sweet things so much? Probably because the only naturally occurring sweet things that our ancestors encountered (fruit, some veggies, honey) were the right combination of good-for-us and rarely available.

And this leads to another opportunity for Big Sugar. It turns out that human taste buds adjust to sugar the way our eyes adjust to the light. This means the more sugar you eat, the less you taste it. In order to get the desired sweetness, you have to add more sugar. As people's taste buds become less sensitive to sugar, they crave more. In other words, the more they add to our food, the more we want it in our food.

One important question to ask when it comes to sugar is: Why does it taste so good when it is so bad for us?

Sweet, for most people, is a pleasurable taste because it was important to our survival. As we have discussed, naturally occurring sweet foods are both rare and seasonal. This combination of *rarity* and *nutritional importance* probably caused our ancestors to evolve increased sensitivity for and enjoyment of sweet tastes.

And they evolved another very important trait that was once lifesaving that is now being exploited by food manufacturers and the sugar industry itself.

Eating sugar stimulates appetite.

When you eat sugar, your body produces insulin, which breaks down sugar quickly. Your body absorbs and/or uses that sugar immediately, and you're left with excess insulin in your bloodstream. That translates into a craving for more sugar. In other words, eating sugar stimulates your appetite for more sugar.

Imagine two of our ancestors, walking through the savanna some 30,000 years ago. It's been a long summer, and berries are showing up on the trees and root vegetables are plentiful.

They stop at a bush and pick a few berries. The berries are sweet and enjoyable. Once their bellies are full, our two early humans move on. A few minutes later, with surplus insulin, they have low blood sugar and suddenly have powerful cravings for more berries. They go back for another batch. And they end up eating until their bellies are distended and full.

Today, this behavior is dangerous, but back then, this was a great idea because as their bodies processed the sugar and ran out of places to store it, they started creating fat; stored calories and water that might be the very things that helped them survive the coming winter.

For eons, this craving for sugar saved our ancestors by boosting their cravings, motivating them to eat more than they needed so that they could fatten up and survive the winter. Now, this very same evolutionary trait is our Achilles heel, and the food industry is using it to drive their profits.

And, to make matters worse—or better for the sugar industry— sugar is both emotionally and physiologically addictive. There are physical withdrawal symptoms, and animal studies have shown the addictive nature of sugar. There's also the emotional addiction of sugar.

Let's go back for a moment to our Paleolithic tree laden with berries. Let's imagine that we've been walking past that bush for three or four weeks, and the berries have been green every time. They've been camouflaged within the green foliage of the plant. They're not advertising themselves. But one day, you and I are walking by and we see that the berries have now turned red. We recognize them for what they are, and we know that they're sweet. Here in the Paleolithic era, we're living in an environment and a social construct where calories are scarce and rare and sweet is even more so. When we see these berries, our hearts skip a beat; we get excited and start producing dopamine and serotonin—before we even eat one.

The same thing happens today when a child sees an ice-cream stand. She knows the treat is going to taste good and be full of sugar. She starts producing serotonin and dopamine before she even gets the ice cream in her hand.

We eat the berries off our tree. She eats her ice cream. The flavor and texture and olfactory experience of eating that fruit or eating that ice cream is linked to, and influenced by, the really positive feelings created by serotonin and dopamine.

People often say that they eat something because it makes them feel good. What actually makes them feel good is the sight of the food, the permission they give themselves to eat it, or simply the rebellious decision to eat something they know they probably shouldn't. They get a boost of serotonin, a boost of dopamine, and then, in an internally drugged state, they eat those foods and the food tastes even better than it really does. They are literally in an internally drugged positive state. Eating foods in that state links those foods to that state. This in turn creates an emotional addiction. As a result, they believe that they can access that same great feeling again by eating that particular food.

Now, food manufacturing companies know they can turbocharge this by adding more sugar to emotionally charged foods. They can really boost that cycle of emotional addiction and couple it to the physical addiction of sugar as well.

So that's what they do.

They use sugar to make food addictive.

They add more sugar to trigger increased appetite and more eating.

They commission research and studies to hide the damage they are doing.

They use manipulative marketing campaigns to link emotions to their foods.

And then they shift the blame for the damage they are doing onto the consumer.

SHIFTING THE BLAME: ACT II

In social anthropology there is a concept associated with levels of civilization called "calories per acre." Nomadic hunter-gatherers live within a sparse landscape that has a very low level of calories per acre, perhaps a few thousand. The Masai, who are pastoralists tending goats and cattle, have a much higher level, hundreds of thousands of calories per acre, because they keep their animals with them. Go up the chain to agriculturalists, and they have millions of calories per acre available to them because they are directly affecting the growth of the plants around them and also keeping livestock.

The next level is civilizations with marketplaces and financial economies where people can trade for calories and don't need to physically acquire them. Fast-forward to America in the 1950s, when people lived in an era of billions of calories per acre. Now, over the last ten years, civilization has "evolved," if we can use such a term, to billions of calories per couch, because now, with Uber Eats and DoorDash and similar services, you need expend no more energy than it takes to walk from the couch to the front door to acquire all the calories you want.

The human instinct to preserve energy is still strong, and it makes us lazy. The food industry has capitalized on this by making food incredibly convenient for us, with drive-through restaurants and packaged food and Happy Meals and on and on. We don't have to expend any energy to acquire food or water during the day. Because of that, we're loading up on absolutely atrocious food and doing very little to burn it off. As a population we have become overweight, unhealthy, and unhappy, and it is only getting worse and spreading around the world.

This epidemic of unhealthiness has put pressure on food companies. Soft drink sales are declining, for example. They're becoming less popular as people change their eating habits to move away from sugar. Over the last 20 years, sales of full-calorie soda drinks have dropped by 25 percent.[3] Soft drink firms began competing with the health food industry and the energy drink industry, the makers of Red Bull and Monster and so on. What did they do in response? Did they make their drinks better, healthier? No. They began lobbying to push people not to change their diets but to exercise more. Coca-Cola announced they were supporting a "science-based" solution to the obesity crisis.[4] Are you surprised to learn that their "science-based" solution found that the way to control obesity did not involve cutting down soft drink consumption? Their "solution" involves more exercise! What a surprise!

A nonprofit called the Global Energy Balance Network (GEBN) was founded to advocate for better health by encouraging more exercise. GEBN supports the proposition that if you are concerned about your weight, you should be exercising more. Steven Blair, the vice president of GEBN, said in a speech announcing the formation of GEBN that "most of the focus in the popular media and the scientific press is, 'oh, they're eating too much, eating too much, eating too much,' blaming fast food, blaming sugary drinks, and so on. And there's really virtually no compelling evidence that that is in fact the cause."

Why would he say something like that? We have to consider the motive. Any business would worry about losing 25 percent off the top—that's a big hit. There's certainly a motive to address that slide on the part of the soft drink companies. But why would an executive at a supposedly independent nonprofit say what Blair said? Consider this: in 2014, Coca-Cola donated $5 million to the organization. Maybe that doesn't mean anything. Maybe it does. Then there's this: the website GEBN.org is registered to Coca-Cola.

The company explained that they registered the site on the organization's behalf, as a favor.

Do you believe that? We don't.

Anyone who's paying attention knows that GEBN is just a lobbying front for the soft drink industry. Such industry-tied organizations are a familiar tool of many industries under scrutiny. Despite the industry's disingenuousness, in one sense their argument is right: People are not moving enough. They're not getting enough exercise. If you want to launch a really powerful propaganda campaign, the best thing to do is build it on just enough truth that it can stand up on its own legs. GEBN went and identified a truth—the average person doesn't get enough exercise—but then took that argument to a different conclusion, asserting that the sole reason for the obesity and diabetes epidemic is that people don't get enough exercise.

Shifting the responsibility onto the consumer is good business; it may serve to provide some protection from costly liability suits similar to those faced by the tobacco industry and allows them to continue selling their disastrous "nonfood" products to unsuspecting consumers.

Similarly, we regard the label "lifestyle disease" as part of this same shameful strategy to shift the blame for their dangerous products onto the consumer. By calling diabetes, obesity, hypertension and other conditions "lifestyle" diseases, they are blaming the consumer for damage caused by their own products and their continual efforts to increase demand for those products.

The truth that they are aiming to conceal is that these epidemics have much more to do with sugar than anything else. Sugar is both dangerous to our health and the lever by which food manufacturers have manipulated our evolutionary adaptations to drive demand for their products.

We are not arguing against exercise; we are all for it. We are simply arguing against the food industry suggesting that getting enough exercise will solve all our health problems. Our position is that *exercise will not make you healthy, but it will make you healthier.*

Further, we suggest that this exercise-your-calories-away campaign has motivated many people to do excessive levels of exercise while malnourished, toxic, and overweight, which has then caused themselves other diseases or injuries.

When Boris Johnson, the prime minister of the United Kingdom, recovered from COVID-19, he publicly acknowledged how dangerous it was for him to be so overweight, and he made two important announcements:

1. He was determined to solve the obesity problems of the United Kingdom.

2. He was moving away from his previously more conservative or libertarian view of food (where people should just make their own decisions) and now understood that government has a role to play in fighting the obesity epidemic.

This sounded good to us. Shortly afterward, we received a note from a consultant working with the British parliament that was familiar with our work. They asked us to draft a letter to Mr. Johnson to offer to help on his "war against obesity," and so we did. A few weeks later, we received word the letter was on the PM's desk.

And so we waited.

While we were waiting, Mr. Johnson announced his strategy for fighting obesity, and guess what? It came straight from the pages of the soft drink industry suggestion that people just need to move more. He was going to bicycle his fat away.

COVID-19 has given every government in the world the ammunition and inspiration needed to make serious food industry reforms, and one by one each government is squandering this chance.

Again, we are all for exercise, provided you are generally healthy and well-nourished first.

As we have discussed, our ancestors were required to move to survive; they were forced to walk, climb, hunt, and dig on a regular basis. Further, the fruits of their movement often came in the form of nutritional windfall. A successful foraging trip might have turned up near gluttonous levels of plant material, and a successful hunting trip might have resulted in more meat than could be eaten in a single day.

Our ancestors were capable of gorging; our stomachs, normally the size of a fist, are well able to stretch and expand to take advantage of these opportunities of abundance. It was a good thing, too, because any one windfall may well have been followed by days, weeks, or even months without such success.

Today we're conditioned to eat three big meals a day, which is not how our relationship with food evolved. Typically, we eat a big sugary breakfast that stretches our stomach out. A few hours later we may be in some sort of mild insulin shock, which causes us to feel groggy, maybe a little spacy, and certainly hungry—and this hunger is exacerbated by the now-empty, still distended stomach. A handful of nuts is not going to satisfy that kind of hunger. The result is a cycle of craving large meals and cramming in more food than we need. (One reason you see a rise in the practice of intermittent fasting among some health-conscious people is because there is a growing recognition that, just like the pancreas, the stomach is not supposed to work the way we ask it to work; it needs a break from time to time.)

Do we get less exercise than we should? Absolutely.

Our ancestors were probably very good energy conservationists; they didn't waste energy on movement that wasn't necessary for some reason. We have a powerful instinct to take it easy, to rest up for whatever might be coming next.

One might say that we are fundamentally lazy, that our instincts tell us to conserve energy. Naturally, we look for the easiest way to get energy. The food industry knows this and works very hard to make food as easy as possible to attain. (Seventy percent of the people who go to McDonald's use the drive-through.[5])

And so, convenience is yet another tool in the food industries' profit-seeking arsenal. They have made the worst possible sugar-rich foods easy, effortless, and convenient. Now, many of us are eating the worst possible foods and doing almost no work to get them.

And so, we are contending with:

- The chemical addiction of sugar and insulin, each of which causes us to want to eat more
- The emotional addiction of foods that trigger feel-good chemicals when we eat them
- The hunger of a regularly distended stomach
- Our evolutionary tendencies toward eating too much
- Our instinct to conserve energy and move the least amount possible.

We've created quite a cycle, haven't we?

In order to solve a problem, it is really helpful to fully understand how it was created. Many years ago, the governments around the world decided that it was important to put together recommended food and nutrition guides to help people make better food and lifestyle decisions.

The U.S. government nearly got it right, but then they made one mistake that might just be the most significant influence in the creation of the current diabetes and obesity epidemics. We will explore that mistake and what we can do about it in the next chapter.

CHAPTER 2

The Intersection of Food, Disease, and Profit

The food industry has been manipulating what we eat, and what we're told to eat, for a long time. If you were born before 1980, you likely remember the four food groups, which were promoted by the U.S. Department of Agriculture. After that came food pyramids promoting how much we were supposed to eat of various foods.

But where did these ideas about how to eat come from?

Let's start with a discussion about food science and food research. Imagine that you got an exotic animal for a pet (clearly not a good idea but important for this example). How would you know what your new wild animal needed for food? Would you scour PubMed looking for research? Would you reach out to the pet food makers to ask their opinion? Or would you, perhaps, tune in to National Geographic and watch a show about your new pet and see how it lives in nature and what its natural diet is?

At the various stages over the last 100 years that food regulations were created, the food manufacturers have played the role of the pet food makers in this example. They have been directly involved, and it is important to know that their primary objective for being involved in those discussions was to preserve (or capture more) market share. They are not interested in our health.

Back to the "four food groups."

The four food groups were first formally developed in the 1950s, although they had been promoted earlier by Kellogg's co-founder W. K. Kellogg. When he noticed that school systems were running low on money, Kellogg offered to print up really beautiful color posters they could hang in their buildings that promoted what he called the four food groups. Prior to the development of these posters, grain was really a dietary afterthought. Yet with the advent of the four food groups, suddenly 25 percent of the plate was to be covered by grains. Kids grew up believing in the idea of the four food groups and that a balanced diet had to include pasta or bread or some kind of cereal for breakfast.

After the USDA developed a draft of the food groups, the agency invited executives from major food companies to comment on them because they believed those companies would have a "vital interest" in any food guides the government developed. Not surprisingly, those executives agreed that they did, indeed, have a vital interest in government dietary recommendations. The executives of Kellogg's, General Mills, C.W. Post, and other companies were invited to the USDA offices to offer their commentary and recommendations.

Suddenly, dairy products were deemed to be an important part of the four food groups. Grains remained a major feature. The four food groups became part of the American psyche, and because of America's international reach, they became internationally understood. People began to talk about a "balanced diet." What was that? Historically, the term has meant that it was a good idea to consume a wide variety of nutritionally important foods. But in the 1950s, we began to think in terms of dividing our plate into slices, with so much plate-space dedicated to this food group and so much dedicated to another food group.

Meanwhile, as we discussed in Chapter 1, there was very clear evidence in the late 1960s to demonstrate that there was a link between excessive sugar consumption and heart disease. That research was buried by the sugar industry, which promoted the idea that fat was the culprit. The next thing you knew, the low-fat movement was kicked off, and everybody took their eyes off sugar. If you look at the growth of diabetes from then until now, it's phenomenal. The link between increased sugar consumption and the explosion of type 2 diabetes is no simple coincidence.

According to the Centers for Disease Control and Prevention (CDC), less than 1 percent of Americans had type 2 diabetes in 1958. Before the end of the 1970s, the percentage had more than doubled. By the turn of the century, almost 5 percent of Americans had become diabetic, and by 2015 that number was almost 10 percent. That is a nearly 1,000 percent increase.

One thing we wondered about the epidemic: Who wins?

We already knew that the food industry was winning by selling more of their nutritionally questionable sugar-rich and addictive foods. But we have to consider the cost of treating 1,000 percent more diabetic patients. The pharmaceutical companies are making a killing.

How did this happen? How did the American people drift so far off course so quickly? How did the government or the CDC let this happen?*

In the 1980s, when it became clear that the four food groups were failing to promote good health, Luise Light, Ed.D., was recruited by the USDA from her teaching job at New York University to develop a new food guide. It was to be a good guide that would help America correct course, prevent needless personal suffering, and save the healthcare system millions of dollars.

She and her team created the guide and submitted it to the USDA for approval. When they got it back from the USDA, they were dismayed. The new and official Food Guide Pyramid was completely different from the one they had designed. Light commented that, "The health consequences of encouraging the public to eat so much refined grain, which the body processes like sugar, was frightening." She went on to say, in an article she wrote in 2004, "I vehemently protested that the changes, if followed, could lead to an epidemic of obesity and diabetes."[1]

---

* This story comes from *A Fatally Flawed Food Guide* by Luise Light, Ed.D. (2004) and "Sold to the Highest Bidder—the Fatally Flawed Food Pyramid" by Jon Herring.

Light's original recommendations sought to reduce the consumption of poor-quality carbohydrates, but the altered version recommended quantities 300 percent to 400 percent higher than she had. Equally, she sought to increase people's intake of fresh fruits and vegetables yet found that her recommendations had been reduced by 60 percent.

Further digging led to understanding. Her guide—a guide that would surely have saved lives and reduced the strain on the medical system—was handed over to USDA advisors before being made public. It took 12 years for her guidelines to reach the public. By the time they did, the health and well-being of Americans had been sold to the highest bidders: the various food industry lobbyists that stood to lose if her guidelines were published as she designed them. The changes made to her team's original design were the work of special interest groups attempting to preserve or increase their plate-share without any consideration for the personal suffering or public cost of their intervention.

We are forced to ask why the USDA (United States Department of *Agriculture*) was even responsible for creating food guidelines; surely the surgeon general's office might have been a more appropriate and objective team?

The USDA and their industry advocates didn't stop at changing the food guidelines. They also changed the recommendations to include "meaningless—even deceptive—recommendations," Light tells us, such as "choose carbohydrates wisely for good health" and "choose fats wisely for good health."

This ambiguous language has proved both dangerous and costly, as the rise in obesity and diabetes proves. The personal suffering this has created is immeasurable, and the cost to the public purse is in the billions.

Further, Light wrote that the government didn't want to make any foods off-limits, so the new and improved guidelines included "discretionary calories" from added sugar and fats without comment on the quality or type of sugar or fats.

Now, as we look back over the last 25 years, it is clear that Light's predictions of epidemic levels of diabetes and obesity have come to pass.

In the book *Making Healthy Places*, the authors pointed out how serious the situation had become:

> [Obesity's] prevalence has increased with a striking rate since the 1960s, when an estimated 45% of Americans were overweight or obese. Now, two out of every three American adults 20 years or older are overweight or obese.
>
> Before 1985, among the states with data available, no state reported an adult obesity prevalence higher than 15%. In 2009, only one state—Colorado—had an obesity prevalence of less than 20%.
>
> Since 1970, the prevalence of obesity among U.S. children and adolescents has tripled. Between 1970 and 2008, obesity rates in 6- to 11-year-olds have risen from 7% to 20% and for adolescents, from 5% to 15%.[2]

Since then, the situation has only become more serious. According to an NCHS data brief in February 2020,[3] obesity rates in the United States have increased by 30 percent between 2000 and 2018, and severe obesity rates have doubled during that same time period to an incredible 9.2 percent of the adult population.

The impact of these trends is both devastating to quality of life and puts undue pressure on our healthcare systems around the world.

As of this writing, COVID-19 has infected almost 771 million people and caused 6.9 million deaths worldwide and 1.1 million deaths in the United States. By comparison, diabetes, the seventh-leading cause of death in the United States, causes roughly 85,000 deaths *every single year* in America alone.

Another interesting perspective is that COVID-19's "death per 100,000 people" rate in the United States is 25.71 according to Statista.com. Interestingly, diabetes also has a deaths per 100,000 rate of 25.7, according to the CDC.[4] As close as these numbers are, there are two very important differences:

1. The diabetes number happens every single year.

2. Diabetes and obesity appear to be a major influence in the outcome of a COVID-19 infection.

While, at the time of this writing, the data related to the COVID-19 pandemic is still coming out, it is becoming quite clear that preexisting diseases play a major role in how well people fare when infected by COVID-19.

The *Daily Mail*[5] reported on a study done in Italy that demonstrated that 99 percent of those succumbing to COVID-19 had at least one other major disease and that 48.5 percent of those people had three or more other major diseases.

Another study[6] in the New York area found that 88 percent of those hospitalized with COVID-19 had two or more comorbidities.

The mortality rate for COVID-19 is heavily influenced by the underlying health of the patient and therefore by nutrition-related regulations and legislation. OurWorldinData.org reviewed case fatality rates of COVID-19 in China and found that mortality rates appear to be heavily influenced by preexisting conditions, including diabetes.

The COVID-19 mortality rates[7] for people with preexisting diseases appear to as follows:

- 10.5 percent for those with cardiovascular disease
- 7.3 percent for those with diabetes (and diabetes contributes to all these other conditions!)
- 6.3 percent for those with chronic respiratory disease
- 6 percent for those with hypertension
- 5.6 percent for those with cancer
- 0.9 percent for those without a preexisting condition

This means that a person with diabetes is 800 percent more likely to die from a COVID-19 infection than a person without a preexisting condition.

This early data leads us to the believe that that preexisting good health is the best defense against a pandemic like the one caused by COVID-19 and that the changes made to Light's Food Guide Pyramid might be among the most significant factors in the severity of the COVID-19 pandemic.

When we couple this information with the explosion of diabetes and obesity in America and around the world over the last 30 years, we are forced to ask if the sugar industry had not captured the 20 percent of the plate calories lost to fat, would COVID-19 even have caused a pandemic?

Since it appears that as much as 90 percent of COVID-19-related hospitalization and death is caused by these preexisting, generally food-related diseases, it is our contention the entire pandemic could have been avoided if the food manufacturing, marketing, and lobbying industry had been brought to heel in the 1950s.

In fact, we would go so far as to suggest that if sugar had not devastated the underlying health of the world's population, the Great Lockdown of 2020 would never have happened.

This may seem like a strong statement, but when you compare case fatality rates and co-morbidities, it seems fair to suggest that, without prolific diabetes and obesity, there would have been 90 percent fewer hospitalizations and death and, therefore, no need for lockdowns.

Given this, it makes sense that the governments around the world would want to provide accurate food, health, and nutrition guidelines. Where it got tricky was when they allowed large food manufacturers to influence their recommendations. Before COVID-19, some countries were already starting to see the light and had begun changing their food guidelines. Notably, Sweden, while still slow to adopt the guidelines at a national level, has confirmed that data from 16,000 studies indicate that a low-carbohydrate and higher (healthy) fat lifestyle can be very effective for people suffering from obesity or diabetes.

Canada, whose food guides have for many years been very dairy-industry influenced, received recommendations in 2018 from Health Canada that they should issue warning labels on certain food items, including dairy products. In 2019 the official Health Canada food guide all but dropped dairy products.

Countries are catching on; a healthy population is a population that places much less stress on healthcare systems and healthcare workers.

Perhaps, with all the data coming out of the COVID-19 pandemic, governments around the world will see how important it is to get the food guidelines (and resulting regulation, education, taxation, and legislation) out of the hands of profit-seeking food manufacturers and lobbyists and into the hands of nutritional scientists.

While it is easy to place blame at the hands of food manufacturers and lobbyists, it is also important to understand our own roles and responsibilities in creating these circumstances. In the next section, we will discuss cravings, food reward systems, and how we trained the food industry to treat us this way.

THE INCENTIVE TO ACT BADLY

Humans evolved cravings for foods that were both nutritionally important and rare. If something was nutritionally important and readily available, you didn't need to evolve a craving for it; general hunger would be enough to make sure that you got what you needed.

But if something was nutritionally important and rare, our ancestors may have required motivation beyond hunger to seek that something out. Take fruit, for instance: full of vitamins, minerals, and energy but only available for a few days or weeks at a time. Without a powerful craving for it, we might not even notice that fruit was in season, and we may then miss out on badly needed nutrients and energy.

Further, our bodies have reward systems; when you eat a piece of fruit, the body rewards you with feel-good chemicals like dopamine. This teaches you to keep an eye out for it when it comes back into season.

These cravings and reward systems evolved over periods of time during which fruit was seasonal and small. The cravings and reward systems create an almost addictive desire for the food, making sure that we get as much as we can before it is all gone. As we have discussed, this may well have been lifesaving for our ancestors because eating all that fruit in the late summer or fall would help them to fatten up for what might become a very long, drought-filled winter.

Today, fruit (and its distant but damaging cousin, refined sugar), is so common that this craving/reward system has become dangerous. The average American now eats 156 pounds of sugar every year, compared with an average consumption of only 4 pounds in 1700, 18 pounds by 1800, and 60 pounds by 1900.[8]

Further, this craving/reward system is widely abused by those in the food manufacturing industry who force cheap carbohydrates into our food. Take a look at any name-brand tomato sauce on the grocery store shelf. Turn it over and read the ingredient list. Ingredients are listed by volume; sugar will be the second- or third-highest ingredient. Why would it be there? Any chef who knows what they are doing will tell you that you need a pinch of sugar to balance the acid in the tomatoes, and they'd be right. But you don't need so much sugar that it is the second- or third-highest ingredient. That much sugar creates insulin spikes, which translate into sugar cravings. Suddenly you're ordering seconds. Or thirds. And the more food you're eating, the more profit that tomato sauce-making company is earning.

We are not saying there are evil people working in the food industry or the pharmaceutical industry. Most people working in those businesses believe they are doing good work. Unfortunately, in the capitalist system in which we live, there are rents and taxes to pay and investors who want a return. That creates an inexorable pressure to make money.

This pressure affects all businesses, including those in the food and pharmaceutical industries. We've seen what profit-seeking in the food industry has done; let's take a look at the pharmaceutical industry and how they have approached diabetes.

An Ancient Disease

Diabetes itself is not new. We've known about it for a long time. The ancient Romans knew when one of their soldiers had diabetes because their urine on the ground, full of sugar, would attract ants. What's different is that over the last 30 or 40 years, diabetes has become an incredibly profitable disease.

The American Diabetes Association says that someone diagnosed with diabetes faces about $16,000 in annual medical costs. About $10,000 of that is for treatment.

When Rubén was in medical school, every Wednesday was "drug day," and the pharmaceutical representatives made presentations to doctors passing by their booths about their latest wonder drugs. They'd invite doctors and students to dinner presentations and sporting events. They constantly offered freebies. Rubén felt like he was being trained to be a "drug pimp." He learned how to identify diseases, the constellation of things happening in the body associated with that disease, and which medication to recommend. Those pills and injections were not only expensive but also had a lot of side effects, so Rubén also learned how to treat those too.

The *British Medical Journal* reported that the pharmaceutical industry paid out around $600 million to healthcare professionals and organizations in the United Kingdom in 2016.[9] About two-thirds of those professionals or organizations disclose the payments they receive, but "some of those doctors who receive the bigger payments have withheld their names, as they are entitled to do."

In the United States, an investigation by ProPublica found that, between 2009 and 2013, 17 pharmaceutical companies paid out over $4 billion[10] to increase prescription rates by doctors. The payments come in the form of speaking fees, consulting, meals, travel, and royalties. Over a five-year period, thousands of doctors received over $100,000; more than 2,500 received at least $500,000; and 700 doctors received over a million dollars. A few startling examples include, according to the ProPublica report, $29 million for Kevin T. Foley (neurological surgery), $10.5 million to Gail S. Lebovic (plastic and reconstructive surgery), and $6.25 million for Gary Carr (dentistry).

The ProPublica investigation revealed some specific promotion campaigns, including $17.9 million to promote Xarelto (a blood thinner), $12.2 million to promote Humira (an immunosuppressant), and $12.6 million to promote Farxiga (a diabetes drug).

These numbers may seem large, but Farxiga brought drugmaker AstraZeneca $835 million in 2016 and then posted a 28 percent increase in sales in 2017. We are talking about billions of dollars.

It is also worth noting that, according to the *British Medical Journal*, there appears to be an inverse relationship between the budget to push the drug and its effectiveness. Drugs that are marketed with physician-promotion payments are "less likely than top-selling and top-prescribed drugs to be effective, safe, affordable, novel, and represent a genuine advance in treating a disease."

In other words, drugs that "work" appear to market themselves, but drugs that are less effective and less safe need millions of dollars of extra push to gain market acceptance.

For example, the FDA has issued warnings about Farxiga (despite approving it in 2014), including that use may lead to "conditions that can be fatal."

Plaintiffs in a number of lawsuits against drugmakers Astra-Zeneca, Bristol Myers Squibb, and Johnson & Johnson claim that these manufacturers knew that Farxiga (and Invokana) were potentially dangerous and that they concealed this information from both doctors and patients.

Drugwatch reports that "plaintiffs' injuries include amputations, kidney damage, diabetic ketoacidosis, and a flesh-eating disease called Fournier's gangrene. As of April 2019, there were 965 Invokana lawsuits and 37 Farxiga lawsuits pending in federal courts."

Luckily, prescribing drugs for diabetes is not the only option.

The Tale of Two Bantings

William Banting, born in 1796, was obese, something that was very rare in the late 1800s. Concerned about his weight, he consulted his physician, Dr. William Harvey, who suggested that Banting try a diet that he had learned about for diabetes management.

Dr. Harvey had attended some lectures in Paris by Claude Bernard. Bernard was a French physiologist who did groundbreaking work and laid the foundations for understanding homeostasis (optimal functioning of the organism). I. Bernard Cohen, of Harvard University, called Bernard "one of the greatest of all men of science."

Banting managed to reverse his obesity and was the first to popularize the idea of carbohydrate restriction for weight management. In 1863, he wrote a booklet that detailed all the "diets" and treatments he had attempted and then he shared what had finally worked for him; his plan emphasized avoiding sugar, saccharine matter, starch, beer, milk, and butter. The pamphlet became a book, and the book generated significant profits, all of which he donated to charity.

William Banting lived until he was 82 years old, a striking achievement during a time when the average life expectancy was only 48, something he most surely would not have achieved had he not turned around his obesity, which is, statistically, much more dangerous than smoking.

While Banting's diet was incredibly popular at the time and echoed the findings of his physician—that a great many apparently unrelated diseases were actually the result of "corpulence" (obesity)—it would be overshadowed by a discovery by a distant relative of William's some 13 years after his death, Frederick Banting.

Sir Frederick Banting was born in 1891 and was a Canadian medical scientist and physician. In 1923 he was awarded, along with John James Maclead, the Nobel Prize in Physiology or Medicine for his work in the discovery of insulin.

Frederick Banting was also interested in diet, nutrition, and its role in health. Famously, his off-the-record remarks about early fur traders spreading the flu to native Canadians were printed in the *Toronto Star* and included his observation that the trade relationship was doubly unfair. First, he noted that for furs worth $100,000 (fox skins), native Canadians were receiving only goods worth $5,000. Secondly, those goods altered the diet of native Canadians, introducing them to "flour, biscuits, tea, and tobacco," which, he pointed out, caused the death of indigenous residents by supplying the wrong kind of food.[11]

Both the Hudson's Bay Company and the Department of the Interior were unimpressed by his comments, with the former demanding a public retraction. Banting acknowledged that the reporter betrayed his trust by printing his off-the-record comments but refused to retract them; instead he maintained his position in his report to the Department of the Interior.

He warned that the conversion from "race-long hunter" to "dependent trapper" was the gravest danger facing these native Canadians. Specifically, he pointed out that "white flour, sea-biscuits, tea, and tobacco do not provide sufficient fuel to warm and nourish." He also noted that infant mortality was high because mothers were undernourished by this "white man's food" and that, further, he was concerned that tuberculosis had appeared and that a flu-like epidemic had killed a significant portion of the population at Port Burwell.

Did he know, at that time, that the native Canadian people were already following a William Banting–style diet before the Europeans arrived? And that it was moving off that diet that was causing them so much illness and disease?

But the story of the two Bantings has an additional twist.

William Banting proved and popularized the concept of carbohydrate restriction—what we at WILDFIT call Spring or what you may have seen referred to as low carb or keto. His concept was very successful, and he donated the profits to charity.

Frederick Banting's pioneering work with insulin created a drug-based treatment that he sold to the University of Toronto for $1, claiming that his discovery belonged to the world, not to him. He had hoped that by doing so he would make insulin widely available to the people who need it most.

So neither Banting was in it for the money; they both gave their concepts away.

But then what happened? Greed. Ninety percent of the world's insulin demand is met by three insulin providers: Eli Lilly, Novo Nordisk, and Sanofi. These companies use "pay for delay" agreements to keep generic insulin off the market; they pay would-be insulin manufacturers not to produce insulin and keep the market for themselves. And when pay-for-delay doesn't work, the multibillion-dollar providers simply sue the would-be providers into oblivion, protecting their near monopoly.

These companies also have extensive legal budgets and armies of lawyers working to "evergreen" their patents so that they can maintain their monopoly. Sanofi, for instance, makes Lantus (insulin) and increased their price 24 percent from 2016 to 2018. They filed over 70 patent applications seeking to extend their insulin monopoly for another 37 years.

Lobbying has played a major role in preserving market control. The Pharmaceutical Research and Manufacturers of America (PhRMA) spent $25.4 million lobbying the U.S. Congress in 2017.[12] Remember, this is not advertising spend. This is money spent to sway politicians in their favor, to enact regulations and legislation that protect and increase their profits.

The global market for insulin is growing rapidly as food quality continues to degrade. ResearchandMarkets.com reports that the global insulin market was valued at $24 billion in 2018.

And this is just insulin. Sales for Glucophage XR (now generically metformin) were $918 million annually in 2016.

But even more striking is one very powerful truth: *the vast majority of type 2 diabetes (which accounts for 95 percent of diabetes cases) is fully avoidable and reversible and should not require medication.*

This does raise a very important question: why did medication become popular as a treatment for diabetes, rather than the Banting diet?

We believe the answer comes down to two things. One, the diet that Banting created required a lot of personal effort from people. They would have to change their shopping and food preparation habits. They would have had to use willpower to overcome their cravings for sweet things. And that's a problem. Willpower is notoriously unreliable over the long term.

Two, it's just not very profitable to get people to eat differently. (After all, there was never a "nutrition day" at Rubén's medical school during his four years as a student and subsequent three years of internal medicine residency, but there was a "drug day" every week—fifty-two weeks of the year, from 8 A.M. until noon, for seven years.)

As we have discussed, there is a ton of profit in selling people insulin and diabetes-related medications. Imagine a patient sitting in a doctor's office. He gets a diabetes diagnosis. The doctor can prescribe an ongoing regimen of pills or shots, most of which is probably covered by insurance and may well result in a kickback of some kind to the doctor or their clinic. The insurance company makes money. The drug company makes money. Even the doctor might make money. And the patient feels better. It's very good for the patient and very good for the economy. Except that it's not: over the long term it is devastating to the patient, places an incredible strain on the healthcare system, and drives insurance rates sky-high.

The two Bantings created a fork in the road that offered two different ways of treating diabetes. One is highly profitable and takes responsibility away from the patient. The doctor says, "Look, we'll inject you, and you're going to be fine." The other says, "Okay, you'll need to give up some of your favorite foods, go on a diet, and be miserable, but you can beat this thing."

At the end of the day, we took the insulin and medication path. And this was incredibly profitable for the pharmaceutical industry. Was this manipulation, in the way that adding sugar to spaghetti sauce to take advantage of your evolved tendencies is manipulation? Perhaps. But like all businesses, pharmaceutical companies wanted to sell as much of their product—in this case, diabetes medications—as they could. So what did they do?

As we have discussed, "evergreening patents," price fixing, lobbying, and paying competitors to stay out of the market have played an important part. But they also found a way to expand their market.

Commercial organizations are always looking for ways to increase revenue and profits. Typically, the ways to do so are to either increase the number of clients or increase how much the average client spends—for example, by increasing the buying frequency, by increasing the value of what they buy, or by selling them other products. And anyone in business finance will tell you that the best kind of revenue in the world is recurring or subscription-based revenue—like medicines for chronic diseases.

We imagine a group of pharmaceutical executives wondering how they could sell more metformin or more insulin. The only tool available to them is to increase the number of people taking those medications—after all, a patient who is already taking them

doesn't need to take more. (Although, they are told to "simply inject" when they want to have a treat.)

Here's how we imagine the conversation went:

*"The only area where we could really increase sales is among
the 25 percent of Americans who are walking around with diabetes undiagnosed. We could get them to take our drugs and
increase profits."*

"How do we get more diagnosed?"

*"We could put blood-testing kiosks in malls, create scare cam-
paigns, things like that."*

*"Wait a minute. I have another way. What if we gave people
those drugs prophylactically, before they're fully type 2? We
could do it earlier."*

"How do we do that?"

*"We create a new classification called 'prediabetic.' Once some-
one is considered prediabetic, their doctor could determine
whether they should start taking drugs. Since many people will
spend two, three, four, even ten years in a prediabetic condition
before they get to full-blown diabetes, we might get an extra five
or ten years' worth of pharmaceutical consumption."*

*"But surely if they are prediabetic they should be making lifestyle
changes to prevent themselves from developing type 2 diabetes?"*

"Not if we get to them first."

This is, of course, an imagined conversation. But while we see
prediabetes as a warning, a chance to get back on track, the drug
industry sees it as "presales" or market expansion.

After all, there are now close to 100 million people in the
United States that are prediabetic and therefore eligible for medical intervention. That is a very large expansion of the market and
a great opportunity for the manufacturers of insulin and other
diabetes-related medications.

If people were being diagnosed as prediabetic ethically, in a
socially responsible manner, a doctor would look at the trends in

their A1C test results and other indicators, and they would have a frank conversation.

What Is Prediabetes?

Someone can be diagnosed with prediabetes if their blood sugar level is higher than it should be but not quite high enough for a full diabetes diagnosis. Doctors may also refer to this condition as "impaired fasting glucose" or "impaired glucose tolerance."

People who develop type 2 diabetes will generally go through a period of prediabetes, which is often symptom free.

"Listen," the doctor would say, "you're prediabetic. If you don't make some meaningful changes in the way you live your life, you're likely to become a type 2 diabetic. Let me tell you what that means. It means the likely and eventual early loss of your eyesight and possible limb amputation, circulatory problems, and a variety of other health implications. And a shorter life. To avoid that fate, here's what you need to change in your life."

Instead of saying that, most doctors say something like this:

"You're prediabetic. Do you want to go on a diet, or would you rather start taking medication?"

Of course, more often than not, the patient opts for the easy path because, well, it is easier and because most people don't understand that a type 2 diabetes diagnosis can be every bit as serious as a cancer diagnosis.

There is another problem. Calling it "pre" diabetes suggests a certain inevitability; that this is the stage "before" you develop diabetes.

Instead, we would like to suggest that we see type 2 diabetes and prediabetes differently. For one thing, as we have already suggested, we would ask you to consider type 2 diabetes as a recoverable disease or, perhaps, a repetitive stress injury from which you can heal. Secondly, that prediabetes be seen as a warning stage, not an inevitable slide toward full-blown type 2 diabetes.

Seeing Diabetes as an Injury

There is growing acceptance in the medical community that, with the exception of trauma, diseases caused by pathogens, or genetic conditions, most of what we consider diseases today are in fact evolutionary responses to some level of imbalance or some sort of stimuli. We classify most of these diseases as "lifestyle diseases."

In many instances, cancer, for example, can be related back to lifestyle. Lung cancer is often a product of the body processing all the toxins and damage associated with smoking. If someone stops smoking, the body stops having to process those toxins, and that might prevent them from developing cancer or to potentially turn it around.

The body is incredible, and it is constantly working to protect us, sometimes even from ourselves.

If you work in the garden all afternoon raking leaves and you don't wear gloves, you will get blisters on your hands. Some of those blisters may break. If you keep doing this, over time you'll develop calluses. We don't see the blisters or the calluses as *diseases*; we see them as the body doing what it's supposed to be doing in response to how we are living. A callous is a growth, a thickening of the skin due to prolonged or repetitive friction against the skin. It is not a disease; it is the body responding to stimuli and doing its best to protect you.

When Eric saw how quickly some of his clients recovered from type 2 diabetes, he thought about the two Bantings: Frederick Banting, the discoverer of insulin, and William Banting and his diet that prevents and even "cures" diabetes.

And then it dawned on him: perhaps we were looking at diabetes the wrong way. It isn't a disease. It is an injury, a repetitive stress injury, an injury caused by sustained abuse or misuse of the pancreas over time. Like a strained ankle, a strained pancreas can't do its job very well.

If you want to heal your ankle, you give it rest, therapy, and the right support. The more you take care of it, the more likely it will recover. What if we did the same thing for a pancreas? Would the pancreas recover? The anecdotal results that we've both seen again and again indicate that it often will and that the recovery can happen in substantially less time than it took to cause the damage in the first place.

And so we look at diabetes as an injury rather than a disease. We think about it as being treatable and reversible. Such a thing is possible, in the way that climbing Mount Kilimanjaro is possible—one step at a time.

You may think, *Sure, those things are possible. But how practical are they?* To answer that, let's turn the question around and ask how practical it is *not* to turn your diabetes around.

Diabetes cost America around $327 billion in 2020.[13] But those are just statistics. Diabetes is deeply personal for every individual inside that statistic. If you have type 2 diabetes, there are the social and family costs of living a restricted and unwell life. You face the personal cost of having to take medication constantly. You face the risk of a worsened future, high morbidity, and reduced happiness and quality of life. From where we stand, it is completely impractical not to turn your diabetes around and *become postdiabetic.*

What Is Postdiabetes?

Postdiabetes is a medical condition wherein the patient who was once in the diabetic or prediabetic range (A1C, blood sugar) is now displaying improved metrics ranging from the prediabetic to nondiabetic range and trending in that direction.

While postdiabetics will, for a time, have metrics similar to those seen in prediabetics, the trend is the important factor, and that trend should suggest a different course of treatment. In time, a postdiabetic may have numbers in the "normal range" but should remain vigilant about their lifestyle to avoid a return to diabetes and to continue to repair the damage that may have been done while in the diabetic range.

How possible is it? In most cases it is entirely possible. While it may take longer to repair some of the damage that was done during the diabetic period, many people with type 2 diabetes will be able to transition to postdiabetes within a few months. Extreme cases may take a year or more, but it absolutely can be done. In fact, as a testament to the healing power of our bodies, you can reverse diabetes in a much shorter period of time than it took to create the injury in the first place.

You might wonder, if reversing diabetes is so easy, why isn't everyone with diabetes doing it?

Because most people don't know what you've just learned. They don't know it's possible because, in truth, most doctors don't know it's possible. Doctors are not taught that diabetes can be reversed. They are trained to medicate patients for life. You are at the cutting edge of learning a different approach to diabetes: it is an injury that can be treated through lifestyle, just as a sprained ankle can be treated.

Further, people (including many doctors) don't really understand how serious type 2 diabetes is. They see it as an inconvenience that might involve drugs or injections rather than being the first stage of a complex degradation of the body that may result in circulatory problems, heart disease, eyesight loss, limb amputation, and a dramatically increased susceptibility to infection. (For example, at the time of this writing, it appears that diabetes creates a substantial amount more risk of death than COVID-19; diabetics are 10 times more likely to succumb to the disease.)

People just don't understand. Take this conversation Eric had with his mother when she read an early version of this chapter.

"I just had lunch with some old friends, and one of them offered a newly discovered recipe: Pillsbury dough cooked in muffin tins with chocolate inside them and a marshmallow on top. As an aside, she tells us she is diabetic and so she avoids eating fruit, but when she wants an extra 'treat' like the one she just described, she just takes some extra insulin."

This attitude is not my mother's friend's fault; it is how she has been educated about her diabetes. Perhaps if she fully understood the consequences (and that the condition was reversible), she might be open to making some changes.

We should add here too that this is not the fault of doctors. Consider how they have been let down; they can invest thousands and thousands of dollars and years of their lives to learn how to help people and not be required to attend a single class about food or nutrition. And much of their initial and continuing education is funded by pharmaceutical companies. The problem is not doctors; it is a medical system that profits from treating disease instead of preventing it.

In the rest of this book, we will show you how you can change your experience of diabetes. To make these changes, there are times you will have to rely on willpower, and sometimes you will have to go against your instincts. This is because of something Eric calls "the evolution gap."

THE EVOLUTION GAP

For our species, most of our genetic (physical and psychological) evolution took place in response to, or in partnership with, our environment. When our ability to innovate accelerated faster than our genetic evolution, a gap opened. This gap is now responsible for most of our stress, disease, and suffering. That gap is called the Evolution Gap.

Farming, or the intentional cultivation of crops, appears to have originated in at least 11 different locations starting about 12,000 years ago. With the advent of agriculture, we created a change so rapidly that our genetic evolution was not able to keep pace. Our invention and advancement of new social structures and technology opened a gap between our genetic evolution and our environmental realities—the Evolution Gap. The pace of social and technological change is accelerating exponentially and with that, so is the Evolution Gap.

As far as our bodies are concerned, it's still tens of thousands of years ago. The cravings that we have are cravings we developed as evolutionary advantages in a time when food was seasonal, rare, and required significant effort to attain.

Our ancestors evolved a number of traits that served them incredibly well for most of human history but are now causing us significant difficulties and health implications. For instance, our ancestors evolved the following traits:

- Powerful cravings for sugar (seasonal fruits and hard-to-obtain honey)

- Insulin production that stimulates further sugar cravings and fattening up for winter

- Energy conservation—don't waste energy by moving more than necessary

- The easy conversion of sugar to fat to aid in the survival of droughts and food shortages

- Reluctance to release fat particularly when faced with calorie restriction or stress

Each of these traits served our ancestors very well during the time in which they lived, but these traits are no longer serving us; they are now causing incredible pain, disease, suffering, and social cost.

Remember that our powerful cravings for sugar make it difficult for many people to avoid sweet-tasting foods. Our insulin production system was designed to make sure that we ate as much sugar as possible because it was rare, and occasional gorging when possible may have aided in survival during hard times.

In other words, we have genetic traits that may once have been lifesaving but are now incredibly dangerous if we don't apply our intelligence and consciousness to the equation.

Essentially, each of us has an internalized and outdated shopping list and an outdated life coach telling us how we are supposed to live. As you have seen, the food industry is more than happy to take advantage of this Evolution Gap and put sugar in our food to stimulate our appetites.

This is one of the many reasons we are confused; why on earth would God or evolution create things that taste so good but that can also be quite dangerous? And this confusion is exactly what the food industry wants.

COGNITIVE DISSONANCE

The nutrition and diet industries have confused us about food and lifestyle, and they benefit from that confusion. One minute wine is good for you, and the next minute it is bad. Bread is good for you; then you cannot live on bread at all. Or you're told sugar is causing heart disease, whoops, no, it's fat—oh, wait, maybe it's sugar after all.

On November 19, 2020 the *Daily Mail* in the United Kingdom reported on a study using this headline:

"Eating Just ONE Egg a Day Increases Your Risk of Diabetes by 60 Percent, Study Warns"[14]

The article goes on to explain that in a small sample group of entirely Chinese subjects, there was correlation between egg consumption and "high blood sugar levels," but nothing in the study appears to reference the actual development of type 2 diabetes or, for that matter, a causal relationship.

If you look at the actual study, then you will learn some interesting things, including that the correlation between egg consumption and increased blood sugar levels only existed in the female members of the trial and that, interestingly, many of the female members of the trial didn't really like eggs, so they consumed their eggs as *ingredients in baked goods*.

At this stage, I don't think we need a study to tell us that eating muffins, pancakes, and waffles every day with honey, syrup, or jam might cause an increase in blood sugar levels and increase the odds of gaining weight or developing type 2 diabetes. But why attempt to blame eggs for the damage done by grains and sugars with a story that is both dishonest and *intentionally* misleading?

We could speculate as to who might want to push an article that falsely blames eggs for diabetes, but our money is on the sugar lobby. After all, and as we have discussed, they have been caught beetroot-red-handed funding "research" designed to blame fat for the damage caused by sugar.

Oh, and just for fun, here is another headline from the *Daily Mail* a year earlier:

> "One Egg a Day 'Lowers Your Risk of Type 2 Diabetes'; Controversial Study Says It Promotes Fatty Acids That Protect You from the Disease"[15]

And so, people get confused, give up, and simply eat what they want or what they find convenient.

In the coming chapters, we will explore foods that are actually good for you but that should be eaten in certain ways and cycles. We are also going to talk about the role that exercise plays in turning your health around and the fact that for some people exercise is an incredibly bad idea until they have improved their basic health. (As we said in Chapter 1, exercise will not make you healthy, but it will make you healthier.)

We're also going to debunk the popular diet myth that the first thing you should do is eliminate a bunch of foods from your diet. We will introduce you to a new paradigm that says *that your health is far more influenced by you getting enough of the good stuff than by you eliminating the bad stuff.* (Sure, there is some "bad" stuff to consider, but the first step in health is making sure that your body is getting what it needs.)

In the coming chapters, which you'll read week by week, we'll go step-by-step with gradual additions to, and eventual subtractions from, your current diet. We have created a structure that will help you to create lasting lifestyle change that will improve your body's function and your health and reduce the stress on your pancreas so that it can begin to heal.

As you move forward now into Part II of the book, we want to give you some strategies that will help you get the most out of your experience of becoming postdiabetic.

1. Read each chapter week by week; don't skip ahead. (This program follows some of the elements of behavioral change dynamics and is designed to help you create lasting changes without having to use willpower for the rest of your life.)

2. Learn in order to teach. If you go through this book with some idea of who you might share this information with, you will integrate the information much better. When you learn something in order to teach it to someone else, you learn it *deeper*—much deeper. (With whom do you want to share this information?)

3. Journal your progress. Progress is fundamental to human motivation. By recording your journey in writing, you will make it much easier to stick to your plan and create lasting change.

4. Record your numbers. In your journal, keep track of your various health measurements, blood sugar, weight, physical measurements, and your emotional state each day.

5. Find an accountability partner. You can meet other people on this journey by visiting **www.PostDiabetes.com/facebook**.

With those things in mind, we are thoroughly excited to welcome you to the process of becoming *post*diabetic.

PART II

AN EASY-
TO-FOLLOW
9-WEEK PLAN
FOR
REVERSING
DIABETES

CHAPTER 3

Let's Turn This Around

In the previous chapter, we talked about what postdiabetes is and that it is, in fact, achievable in most cases. Postdiabetes is possible even if some of those in the medical community are stuck in the old paradigm that says that type 2 diabetes is a chronic disease* that can only be *managed* and not reversed.

While type 1 diabetes does not appear to be reversible, those dealing with type 1 diabetes can often improve their health and reduce their dependencies on medication.

We covered, in detail, the why; and now we move to the how. In this part of the book, we will share strategies you can use to change your health trajectory and, possibly, reverse your own pre- or type 2 diabetes. Crucially, we will share steps and tactics that require a bit of short-term willpower but help you create a new postdiabetic lifestyle that is easy to stick with and does not require long-term willpower or create feelings of *missing out*.

As your guides on this adventure, we can take one of two approaches to help you get there.

The first approach is simply to give you a set of rules about what you should eat and what you shouldn't eat, about how you

---

* The CDC defines diabetes as a "chronic" disease that affects the way the body turns food into energy. ("What Is Diabetes?," Centers for Disease Control and Prevention, July 7, 2022, https://www.cdc.gov/diabetes/basics/diabetes.html.)

should exercise, and about how you should live. This might work well if you are highly motivated and have very strong willpower. Statistically, however, this system does not work over the long term. Some studies suggest that fewer than one percent of people who go on a "diet" report positive long-term results. And, that many of those one percent rebound or relapse when their willpower finally gives way.

One of Eric's favorite sayings is that "people don't fail diets; diets fail people." And so we will, instead, take the second approach. We're going to take you through a very carefully constructed step-by-step process (with proven efficacy)[†] that's going to work both on your food psychology and your nutrition. You will experience the changes incrementally so that you can create truly *lasting* lifestyle change. You will not only turn around type 2 diabetes but also prevent it from ever coming back.

This section of the book lays out a nine-week transformation program. Over the first three weeks, Phase I, we will work on making very subtle changes to your lifestyle and incredibly deep changes to your psychology. We'll take a look at what you eat, when you eat it, and why you eat it. We'll give you instructions each week for exercises you will do and particular changes you'll make to your lifestyle and your diet.

By the end of Phase I, you will have entered something we call WILDFIT Spring, which you'll learn about in Phase II. In this second phase, Weeks 4 through 6, you'll move your body into a primarily fat-burning metabolism and away from your current sugar-burning metabolism. You will learn about maintaining this metabolism and the benefits of it for your health and for controlling type 2 diabetes.

If you have attempted a keto or low-carb program before, you may see some similarities in WILDFIT Spring—and if you found those programs difficult in the past, please trust the process. Our system and incremental steps really do work.

In Phase III, Weeks 7 through 9, you will learn more about seasonal eating, experiencing Summer, Fall, and Winter, and about

---

† This book has been modeled (with permission) on the structure made famous by WILDFIT90, a program that has an 85 percent success rate and has been the highest-rated program on the Mindvalley platform two years in a row (2018 and 2019).

the benefits of cyclical eating patterns. Your body has been designed to go through different seasons of abundance and lack and is able to buffer nutrients on that basis. By the end of Phase III, you will have a clear understanding of the way the seasons work in concert with your body and how you can use the seasons not only to turn around your type 2 diabetes but also to maintain a healthy lifestyle in the future while enjoying your food a great deal.

Before we move into this nine-week transformation, there are three really important things for you to understand:

1. This absolutely does work in most cases.

2. It is not always easy.

3. Progress is fundamental to motivation.

As we mentioned in the Introduction, it is a great idea to journal your experience and measure your progress. The more you can associate the changes you are documenting to all the progress you are making and improvements you are experiencing, the easier it will be to stick with your plan.

As we move into Week 1 now, here are three concepts we will be working with:

1. Weekly Enhancements: These are transitions or changes you will make each week and might include certain mental processes and/or the adding/removing of certain food items for a time.

2. Self-Talk: You'll tune in to the conversations that you have with yourself every time you eat or think about eating. You will become very aware that you have at least two "food personalities" that tend to argue from time to time; we will help you get them on the same side.

3. The Food Timeline: You'll discover some fascinating things about human reward systems and your relationship with food and sugar. You will finally begin to understand why people eat things that they

wish they wouldn't, and you will take powerful steps toward food freedom.

Making lasting and effective lifestyle change is much easier if you have like-minded people around you, so please join our community at **www.Postdiabetes.com/facebook** and consider engaging a coach if you think that might help you get even better results. Research has shown that having an effective coach can improve your results dramatically. If you would like to have a conversation with one of our trained coaches, please visit **www.PostDiabetes.com/findacoach**.

While our programs have among the highest completion and success rates in the world, it is very clear that people tend to make much better progress when they have a support group and/ or a coach.

CHAPTER 4

Phase I: Food Brain

Are you ready? Let's start your nine-week transformation.

Remember, just read and follow one week at a time and track your progress each step of the way. We are very excited for you because we know where you are headed. After all, we know that postdiabetic is possible.

Note: Remember, too, that this book came with your own unique code for a FREE place in our nine-week coaching program that follows the same schedule as this book. The program is $297 online, but with your special code, you can do the program entirely for free. To find out more, please visit **www.PostDiabetes .com/links/freecoaching**.

Simply use your phone camera to scan this code to automatically visit the page.

WEEK 1

Often, when people want to make substantial changes in their lives—like when they set New Year's resolutions—they aim too high. They try to change too much. They burn out their willpower and fail to establish any momentum.

This journey is not about radical change. This book is not about hitting you with a bunch of strict rules and ridiculous calorie counting. We teach you to make incremental improvements to your psychology and nutrition so that you can create lasting change and feel great about your relationship with food.

> *Eric: The first time I tried to improve my own diet, I struggled like everybody else. I knew what I should eat more of and what I should eat less of. But there always seemed to be a really good reason that "today was different." There were days when I was really productive at work that needed to be celebrated. Then there were the days where I had a really difficult day at work and I needed comfort. Then there was the day my friend was having a birthday with lots of free food, and I didn't want to go without free food. There was the time friends invited me over for dinner and cooked something really delicious that I couldn't turn down. I didn't want to hurt their feelings.*
>
> *What I soon began to find out was that I was very capable, every single day, of coming up with a reason why this was the day that I would make an exception to the way I really wanted to be living.*

We designed this program to help you overcome those very human tendencies. In order to create lasting lifestyle change, we have to understand and then break our emotional eating patterns and do away with all the excuses we have for making "exceptions" on a regular basis.

Our aim is to give you something that we call *food freedom*, which means:

- the ability to eat what you want, as much as you want, whenever you want, without feeling guilt or regret; and

- the ability to NOT eat what you wish you wouldn't eat without feelings of disappointment, regret, or missing out.

This definition may sound counterintuitive, because many people actually *want* to eat things that they wish they wouldn't.

But what if you were able to change *what* you wanted to eat?

What if we were able to help you want to eat really functional foods? What if we were able to help you to not crave the things that are bad for your body and damaging your health?

If we could achieve that, then perhaps we could move toward genuine food freedom, functional health, and long-lasting improvement.

Before You Begin

We know we make progress through measurements, so you should take some! Take some key measurements now and record them in your journal. You want to know how far you have come as you make progress in the following weeks.

Record the following metrics:

HA1C

Blood pressure

Optional: A lipid blood panel and a chem-19 panel to evaluate liver and kidney functions

Weight

BMI

Body fat

Use a tape measure to measure each of these:

Neck

Shoulders

Chest

Arm (bicep)

Midsection

Waist

Hips

Thigh

Inner knee

Calf

Ankle

Mid-program (if not more frequently), take and record your blood pressure and weight.

At the end of the program, record these measurements:

HA1C

Blood pressure

Optional: A lipid blood panel and a chem-19 panel to evaluate liver and kidney functions

Weight

All the body measurements listed above

Instructions for Week 1

As you are reading this sentence, you might have some feelings of nervousness, excitement, or apprehension. Does this program *work*? Will it work for *me*? And you might be preparing yourself for the inevitable feeling of lack as we tell you which foods to avoid.

Before getting to that, let's discuss the schedule. It is easier if you start this program on a Monday, so whatever day you are reading this, don't make any of the changes until the next Monday morning.

That said, let's get right to it. Here are the changes we would like you to make here in the first week of your new life:

Starting this coming Monday, please remove the following foods from your diet . . . actually, this week, remove nothing from your diet. Nothing. In other words, please eat exactly what you were eating last week. *Yes, we are serious.*

This week, we want you to eat exactly what you would eat in a normal week in your life. Specifically:

Do not cut out sugar.

Do not cut out bread.

Do not cut out dairy products.

Do not cut out processed foods.

Do not cut out GMOs.

Do not cut out grains.

You do not need to add any of these things if you were not already eating them, **but it is very important, this week, that you do not try to be** *good* **and cut things out in order to get a head start or speed up the process.**

In fact, as the week progresses, you may well find your cravings or desires subsiding to the point that you don't even want some of the things you normally eat; *please eat them anyway.*

With that clear, please add or increase two things:

Drink lots of water. Drink six to eight glasses of water every day. Ultimately, we are suggesting that you drink about 1.5 to 2.0 liters (6 to 8 cups) per day.

Do some deep breathing every day.

Very often we think our health is determined by what we eat, and there is a huge amount of truth to that, but it is not our only need. Even more urgently than food, we need water. We can live for weeks without food if we have to. We can live days without water. And we can live only minutes without air.

This week, as you begin to become more aware of your psychology around food, we are also going to work on two things that are infinitely more important than food: water and air.

At least three times a day, take a deep-breathing break. While there are many powerful deep-breathing programs, we recommend keeping it simple for now (you can think of it as a cigarette break without the cigarette). Go outside, take a breath in while counting to five, hold that breath at the top for a count of five, and release it for a count of five. Do that five times for each breathing break. (Eric has recorded a breathing exercise* for you that you can watch online.)

Right now, you are probably feeling one of four things, or a combination of them:

1. Thank God. I wasn't ready to give certain things up. I am so relieved.

2. What? This is too easy; this will never work. I want to make some changes right now!

3. A bit of both: confusion. What is going on here?

4. I am already doing these things, and maybe this won't work for me.

If you are relieved, check in with that feeling and maybe make a list of the things you are most relieved not to lose this week. This might be something interesting to share with an accountability partner, the Postdiabetic Community, or your coach.

If you are thinking that this is way too easy and that you want to rush ahead, please don't. As the old expression goes, "If you always do what you always did, you will always get what you always got." This program is different; it works. If you want to get different (say, long-lasting) results, you have to do different things. And so, while this week may seem easy to the point of pointless, please trust us; we know what we are doing.

In this next section, you may even begin to see what we mean.

Listen to Yourself

You may or may not be aware that you often have conversations with yourself about food: debating yourself about what you should eat and what you should not, how much to have and when to stop, and whether or not to have seconds or dessert.

---

* Breathing video by Eric: http://postdiabetes.com/links/5x5breathingbyWILDFIT

This brings up your next project for this week: eavesdropping on yourself. Listen in to your internal dialogue about food. Notice how you talk yourself into exceptions, second servings, dessert, snacks, and treats.

You might find that you have two voices inside your head. At WILDFIT, we call them the Food Angel and the Food Devil.[†] You may notice that they argue with each other. A lot.

You might notice some yummy piece of food, and the Food Devil says, "Hey, I've got to have some of that." And the Food Angel responds, "Yeah, but we're on to another belt hole over here. We need to lose some weight."

The Food Devil says, "You're right about that, but we can make an exception *this time* because we deserve it!"

One of the exercises we want you to do this week is to pay attention to this internal food dialogue. Pay attention to the conversation between your Food Angel and your Food Devil. Listen to how the Food Devil convinces you that *this* is the time you should make an exception. Listen to how the Food Angel argues against that. In particular, pay attention to how the Food Devil tries to manipulate you.

By learning your Food Devil's strategies, you can take their power away. For example, imagine that you were going to buy a car, and before you did, we sat you down and told you what was going to happen.

"Listen," we say, "go talk to our friend who is a car salesman. He's a good guy, but he's going to want to make a commission. Here's what he's going to do.

"First, when you show up on the lot, he's going to come right out of the office, walking tall, with a big smile on his face. He's going to reach his hand out even before he gets to you so he can shake hands. He squeezes just the right amount, looks you in the eye, smiles with his nice teeth, and says, 'Hey, how are you today?'

"That's going to start a conversation between the two of you. He's going to start asking you questions about the past cars you've had and why you purchased them, because that's going to help

---

† Food Angel™, Food Devil™, Sugar Monster™ are Service Marks of WILDFIT® and are used here with permission.

him understand how you've made your past buying decisions. There will come a moment where he points to some cars and offers you different colors and different payment plans. Rather than asking you 'Do you want to buy a car, yes or no?' he's going to ask, 'Red or blue?' He is asking these open questions because they are a more subtle way of leading you into agreement."

Because we've told you about our friend the car salesman, when you arrive on the lot and see him stride out of the office toward you, a little part of you is going to smile and think, "Oh, Eric and Rubén told me he would do that." He's going to stick out his hand, and you're going to think, "Oh my God, it's just like they said."

When he asks you about your previous cars and buying decisions, you're going to notice you feel somewhat reluctant to tell him why you bought cars in the past, because now you know the reason he's asking you. You can see that he wants to gain control so he can manipulate your buying decision. When he finally asks you "Red or blue?" you'll understand the strategy he is using. That will make it a lot harder for him to sell to you.

Use that same sense of awareness this week with your Food Devil. Listen to your own internal conversations. Notice the excuses, the manipulations, the "sales tricks" the Food Devil uses to convince you that *this time* you should make an exception. The Food Devil is going to say things like "Well, wait a minute, it's free!" Or, "You've had such a bad day." Or, "You've been so productive, you deserve a reward!" Or it's somebody's birthday, or your cousin's friend's dog died . . .

If you pay attention to the Food Devil, you'll notice the particular tricks it uses to get you to eat food that the Food Angel would rather you didn't. The more you become aware of those tricks and manipulations, the less power they will have over you.

At first you may have a hard time hearing the dialogue. Maybe your Food Devil is overpowering, and all you hear is, "Go get me that food and eat it," while your Food Angel seemingly doesn't even get a word in. What we want you to know is that you do argue, even if that argument is hard to hear or is very short. That's why it's important for you to listen to and acknowledge the way you make decisions about what you eat. Is there a whisper in the background saying, "No, please don't"? Is there a background murmur that says, "This is going to make you feel bad tomorrow"?

As you walk toward the food, listen deeply. Is there any part of you that regrets what you are doing? If there's even the slightest comment, listen to what the Food Devil says in response. Perhaps your Food Devil is pushy and more vocal than your Food Angel is. In addition to focusing on dialogue, take note of what you are feeling too. Your Food Angel might avoid arguing directly with the Food Devil and instead just feel bad or guilty in the background.

Another way to help you hear the dialogue is to speak it out loud. Say you're going through the airport, you're dehydrated from being on an airplane, and you see a Starbucks. *Mmmm . . . a doughnut with some coffee sounds good.* Whether you decide to get in line depends on the conversation inside your head. Bring it outside and voice it (quietly, under your breath, so people don't think you're crazy!).

"Oh, look, there's a Starbucks!" Listen to what comes next and say that out loud. Perhaps it is, "Do you really want that in your body? Do you really want to put all that caffeine and sugar in? Do you really want to be drinking that?"

If you want to deploy some black belt skills against your Food Devil, grab a journal and write the conversation down like a script, or share them with your accountability buddy or with the Postdiabetic Community.

It might look something like this:

FD: I feel like a snack.

FA: Yeah, but we ate like an hour ago. We are not hungry.

FD: Yes we are. Plus, it will taste so good. And we deserve it.

FA: We agreed to cut down on that kind of thing.

FD: We will, for sure. But not today.

FA: You say that all the time!

FD: I know, but today is special; you really worked hard today and you deserve . . .

We've been collecting scripts from our clients for years,[‡] and some of it is side-splittingly funny—but it's only funny because we recognize similar dialogues within ourselves.

The focus for this week is to pay attention to what the Food Devil says. *Listen* to the Food Devil. And this week, *do what the Food Devil says!* Go ahead and eat that thing you want or that the Food Devil wants.

Because here's the thing. As you become aware of this dialogue, you can begin to resist the Food Devil. You may want the Food Angel to win. You may want to use some willpower. Don't do it. This week, don't try to do anything to be "good" when choosing what to eat, or exercising, than you have done in the past. This week, if the Food Angel is winning the argument, pull out your get-out-of-jail card and say, "Nope. This week it's all Food Devil. Eric and Rubén said so!"

We're not kidding. It's important that you do this, because this week is not an exercise in using your willpower. This week is all about you holding a microphone up to your own food psychology and beginning to understand, perhaps for the first time, what *drives* you to eat, *what* you choose to eat, and *why* you choose to eat it.

We want to underline this point: <u>let the Food Devil win this week</u>.

Many people actually take a step backward this week, because most of the time they are at least *trying* to be good. The Food Angel wins sometimes, day to day. This week, let the Angel lose but only after it puts up a bit of a fight. And then let the Food Devil win. And listen in on the argument. Learn from your Food Devil; how do you talk yourself into eating things that the Angel would rather you didn't?

We want you to eat the way you want, because that is how you are going to learn who you are when it comes to food. Letting the Devil win helps you see what is driving you and what tactics the Devil uses to manipulate you; this is a powerful step in gaining real food freedom.

---

‡ To see some of the food dialogue scripts we have collected over the years, please visit: http://postdiabetes.com/links/foodangel-vs-fooddevil.

The Food Timeline

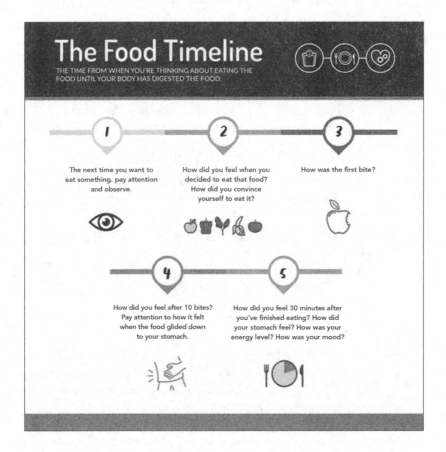

The Food Timeline observes and measures the impact food has on your emotional state of being. Much of what people eat isn't for nutritional sustenance. They eat to change the way they feel. This week, you are going to experience a big difference in your psychology because you have permission to eat the way you want to eat. The reason this is important is when your inner rebel wins, when you say, "Screw it; I'm going to eat what I want," you produce feel-good brain chemicals like serotonin and dopamine.

Here's the kicker: your brain produces those chemicals *before* you eat the food. If you look at the Food Timeline, you will see that people often think that they will feel better eating dysfunctional food, but they actually feel better *before* it goes in their mouth.

When someone makes the decision to, say, eat pizza and ice cream (or berries), the *decision* makes them feel better even before they start eating. This is the trap; it is how bad habits are created and food addition is stimulated.

In essence, it works a bit like this:

Sally ~~Wants~~ NEEDS Chocolate.

Sally is feeling a bit low. A voice pops up in her head and suggests chocolate. Another voice points out that chocolate might not be best since Sally has been trying to "eat better," but in the end, the first voice wins. She rebels against the do-gooder voice and decides to get some chocolate.

At that moment, her body starts producing celebratory chemicals: feel-good internal *drugs* that already lift her spirits even before she eats the chocolate.

Those internal chemicals (dopamine, serotonin) make everything seem a bit better, brighter, and more enjoyable. Including the food. That's right, the chocolate will taste even better because she has these feel-good chemicals in her body. This perpetuates the idea that that chocolate actually made her feel better when it was really the rebellion/celebration.

And then, about half an hour later, she might find that she craves more or that her energy dips. If she eats enough, she might just find that she wakes up feeling puffy and slow the next morning.

This cycle is repeated every day with foods like pizza, soft drinks, chocolate, doughnuts, cookies, ice cream, and many others. And one major problem with this cycle is that Sally, in this case, will separate her memories of the experience so that the feel-good part is linked to eating the chocolate and the consequences are separated by enough time that she will not remember the correlation. In other words, if nonfoods made us feel instantly the way they make us feel later, we would never eat them.

The feel-good *drugs*, produced in the brain as a result of the permission or rebellion, make everything feel, sound, smell, and taste better. A person gives in, grants themselves permission to "treat" themselves, and causes a cascade of feel-good chemicals. Now, feeling good, they smell, feel, and taste the food through the experience of those feel-good chemicals or endorphins. This causes three major problems:

1. It makes the food feel, smell, and taste better than it really is, which creates a false memory of how yummy the "treat" really was.

2. The feeling-good state gets linked up to the smell, feel, and taste of the food.

3. The feel-good chemicals that are created by the rebellious decision will also increase with high-calorie food intake and, in the case of endorphins, will act like anesthesia and reduce your awareness of any negative consequences you might experience with certain food (like itchy throat, low energy, overfilled belly, or headaches).

Much the way Russian scientist Ivan Petrovich Pavlov was able to teach a dog to salivate simply by ringing a bell associated with food, but without actually giving the dog food, your body is able to make you feel good simply by thinking about the food you are going to eat. The tricky part of this is that your body believes it was *the food itself* that made you feel good, not the rebellion or the decision to eat it. This consequence-lag is the start of unconscious eating and even food addiction.

This week, by allowing the Food Devil to win, you will find yourself not wanting as much as you normally might, particularly foods that have been treat foods or reward foods for you in the past. You might find yourself sitting in front of a pizza thinking, *I don't really want that. I don't know if I'm really that interested in eating that pizza.* You'll almost certainly still eat it (we want you to), but without the feel-good brain chemicals you associate with it. You're going to smell and taste and feel that food without the filter of those feel-good chemicals. That's going to permit you to find out whether you really like the taste, whether you really like the experience as much as you thought you did. And to experience the results, if there are any, of eating that food without anesthetic endorphins to blunt the consequences.

You might learn quite a lot this week about your mind and your body.

A common experience we hear from clients and patients in this first week is that they really like the first bite of some treat food. And the second, and third. But then they realize that they're just stuffing their face as they continue to eat without even noticing or tasting it anymore.

This may well happen to you. You will make the decision to eat something; the decision won't be as satisfying because, well, you are supposed to eat it. You will taste the first bite. You might like it. But you also might like it a bit less than before. And the second. And the third. And then you may realize that you are now just eating without the pleasure, or at least with much less pleasure.

Another thing you may notice, something that you may not have paid attention to previously, is how you feel an hour, even 45 minutes, after your meal. Many times when we eat dysfunctional foods like burgers, pizza, and ice cream, we feel sluggish later. Tired, worn out—heavy.

Often, we are so distracted by our lives and the endorphins we spoke of earlier that we don't pay attention to or notice that sluggish or icky feeling. We don't acknowledge the discomfort as a consequence of eating nonfood.

If you knew for sure that you were going to feel yucky an hour later and really connected to that feeling before you took the first bite, you might not take the bite.

When choosing to eat emotionally charged food, we do so to change the way we feel. As you become increasingly conscious of the fact that it isn't actually the food itself that makes you feel better—indeed, that the food will make you feel worse—you will find that willpower doesn't have to be part of the equation anymore. You will simply stop wanting that food as much as you did in the past. This might not happen right away, but over the next few days and weeks you might notice that certain foods have less and less of a hold on you. This is the start of food freedom.

Remember, too, that this book comes with FREE access to our video coaching program; to find out more please visit **www .PostDiabetes.com/links/freecoaching**.

Okay. Stop reading now for a week. Please don't move on to Week 2 until you have finished this week. (We recommend reading about the next week on Friday of the current week and using the weekend as a "buffer zone" wherein the enhancements we have recommended are optional, giving you time to shop and prepare for the coming week.) This will also give you an interesting opportunity to learn more about your food dialogue.

1. Celebration: Watch for progress; are you gaining awareness of your food dialogue? Do you notice any reduction in your cravings or food desires? Are you getting to know yourself better?

2. Note from the Doctor: We've told you to go ahead and eat what you want this week as part of the discovery of your awareness and psychology about food. We know that some of you, out of fear of perhaps losing these foods in the future, might overindulge a bit or a lot. That's okay! But now is the time to become very aware of your blood glucose. Hopefully you have an easy-to-use glucometer at home. Get compulsive about checking your fasting glucose at least every morning, more often if you can, and keeping a log. I think you'll be surprised what happens as you progress through the weeks ahead.

3. Tips for Success

    –   Take your measurements, remove nothing from your diet, add water, do the breathing exercises, and pay attention to your food dialogue and the Food Timeline.

– Stick with it! It may be tempting to try to "be good" and cut out or reduce the quantities of certain "bad" foods; please don't. Eat the way you normally would, even if you don't want to. If you want to get different (lasting) results, you have to try different strategies. Read your Week 2 instructions on the Friday of Week 1.

WEEK 2

Congratulations and welcome to Week 2.

By now you've probably been drinking more water than you were drinking before. You've been taking some nice breathing breaks. And you've been learning a lot about yourself, about your Food Devil and Food Angel and the little tricks the Devil uses to get you to eat things that maybe aren't the best for you.

As you paid attention to your Food Timeline, you may have noticed that it is the decision to eat a particular food that makes you feel better, more than the food itself. You may have begun to see how sometimes the food actually makes you feel less than great after you eat it.

Week 1 is all about awareness and laying the foundation for lasting lifestyle transformation.

We hope you're excited for what comes next, because we are going to do something that is different than what you'll read in the average diet book. Diet books have been failing people for decades upon decades because they ask readers to rely on willpower to make changes, and they ask them to remove foods that they are physically and emotionally dependent on from their diet. Since the average person in the Western world is overfed calories and underfed nutrients, as soon as a diet book gets someone to reduce their caloric intake, they experience severe cravings and actual nutritional hunger. That is why most people only last a few days or weeks on any given diet.

And so, continuing with the theme that getting different re-sults requires taking different actions, we will not, again this week, ask you to remove anything from your diet. Instead, we're going to add in, or increase your consumption of, functional foods, and you'll learn about the Six Human Hungers.

Functional Foods

One of our core health principles, and a key principle of WILDFIT, is that your health is far more dependent on you getting enough of the "good" stuff than it is by you eliminating the "bad" stuff.

So many "diets" start with "remove this" and "avoid that." This may, in the longer term, be a good idea, but true health starts with making sure you get your nutritional needs meet.

For example, imagine putting a person on a theoretically per-fect diet. They eat only what they are supposed to eat—no sugar, no additives, none of the things we traditionally consider bad. Theoretically, they'll be healthy. But if we remove one critical component from that diet—say, vitamin C—they will get sick on this otherwise perfectly healthy diet. They will get skin sores and develop scurvy, and eventually they will die. Even though they have never eaten milk chocolate, sugar, pizza, or ice cream, they will die from malnutrition because they are missing a key nutri-tional component.

This week, rather than asking you to cut out a bunch of foods, we want you to continue to eat as you normally do and to add in or increase your intake of functional, healthy foods. This week we will ask you to increase the quantity, quality, and variety of fruits and vegetables in your diet. We are also going to ask you, if you are not vegetarian, to increase your intake of ethically raised and high-quality animal protein like fish, poultry, eggs, and meat.

If you've done some reading about diets, you might object to this prescription. You might have heard that fruit is evil, or wrong, or bad because it contains sugar. Let's think about that for a mo-ment. Our ancestors, whose digestive system we live with today, didn't think fruit was bad. They thought it was delicious. They ate as much of it as they could whenever they found it. But they didn't find it that frequently, because fruit is seasonal. What's bad is overeating fruit over long periods of time. Fruit is healthy as an occasional food.

We're definitely going to add fruit this week, with one rule: it's best to eat fruit on an empty stomach. Fruit and humans have been in a long evolutionary negotiation that basically works like this: The fruit says, "I will provide you with a really high-calorie, high-vitamin, high-nutrient food if you will transport my seeds. In exchange, don't keep those seeds in your digestive tract too long, where they are exposed to destructive digestive fluids and acids."

Fruit evolved to pass quickly through our digestive systems, and when we eat fruit in combination with other foods, we make that more difficult. That often creates problems like heartburn and indigestion.

Our ancestors traditionally ate more than 200 different plant species. Today, the average Westerner eats fewer than 10. Consider increasing not only the quantity and quality of the vegetables you eat, but also the variety. In order to help you do that, we are providing smoothie recipes that you can use to increase your intake of vegetables in a time-efficient way. You can also add in salads, stir fries, and other vegetable-rich meals and side dishes. (We've provided recipes in the Appendix.) Unlike fruit, you can eat vegetables at any time of day and in any combination with other foods. We have also included the recipe for our Alkagizer Smoothie, which is a great way to increase your intake of fruits and vegetables.

You may also be wondering why we are asking you to increase your intake of healthy meats, fish, poultry, and eggs, especially if you are vegetarian. Please take a look at this video by Eric: http://postdiabetes.com/links/flexitarian.

You might be wondering how you can possibly eat all this.

We're not asking you to stuff yourself silly. We do want you to make sure you eat these additional healthy items, *and that you continue to let your Food Devil win.* Here's what might happen: as you take better care of your nutritional needs, you may find that you are not as motivated to eat some of the other foods you traditionally ate. Nevertheless, if the Food Devil wants you to eat something, then eat it. Really. Let him or her win; this week you will have some serious breakthroughs if you let the Food Devil win.

The one exception to this approach may be breakfast. If you're starting your day with fruit on an empty stomach, you may not have space to eat your traditional breakfast. If you find you are reducing or eliminating some of what you normally eat at breakfast time, that's fine. However, for the rest of the day, do the best you can to eat as you normally would while also adding in all the good, healthy stuff we've described here.

The Six Hungers

There are six human hungers—six primary reasons why people are driven to eat. §

The first is **nutritional hunger**. If we are low on particular nutrients, such as fats, vitamins, or minerals, we crave them, which drives a desire to eat. Nutritional hunger comes about when your body senses it is low on nutrients it needs. It's a very good reason to eat! This week, as you increase your consumption of nutritionally rich foods, you'll find your nutritional hunger diminishes. The one challenge with nutritional hunger is that it produces nonspecific or "macro" cravings for sugar, salt, or fat rather than for specific food items. This is probably because our food availability was seasonal for most of our evolution, so food-specific cravings might have been rather pointless; the simple desire to eat was enough to make sure that, over the space of months, we attained the nutrients we required. (This also gives us another clue: if you are having a food-specific hunger, it is probably not about nutrition, or if it is, nutrition is not the only motivation.)

The next five hungers are not real hungers, and we experience them for different reasons.

The second hunger is **thirst**. You may think it odd to consider thirst a hunger, but until about 7,000 or 8,000 years ago, our ancestors didn't have pottery. That meant that when they came upon

§   Please see this video on the Six Human Hungers by Eric Edmeades: www.PostDiabetes.com/links/6Hungers.

water, they drank as much as they could. It also meant that a huge portion of the water they consumed came from the foods they ate. If they were dehydrated, their body sent a message to eat, and preferably to eat something that contained water, which might have included fresh fruits, vegetables, root vegetables, and fresh meat.

Today, most of our food doesn't contain a great deal of water, and we can get water in other ways. Unfortunately, we still have an outdated piece of software that says, "Oh, I'm dehydrated. I'd better eat something." For many of us, that means eating something with very little water—say, a bag of potato chips making us feel more dehydrated and reactivating the old software command to *eat more*.

We short-circuit this old software, and this hunger, by consciously drinking more water, which you've already begun to do. It is not a good idea to wait until you are thirsty to drink; thirsty is too late. Our job is to prehydrate.

The third hunger is **variety**. Go out with a group of friends and pay attention as people try to decide where to eat. Someone will say something like, "We could go for sushi," and someone else will say, "Oh, I had sushi yesterday; let's do something else." People tend not to want to eat the same food for two or three days in a row.

We think of this as an evolutionary throwback. Our ancestors would have eaten with the seasons and may have found themselves eating a limited variety of foods for an extended period of time. The desire for variety would eventually kick in to make sure that they were getting all their needs met and not just going with easy-to-obtain food. The hunger for variety was a hunger for balanced nutrition, and it pushed our ancestors to move to other locales or otherwise change up their diet. For instance, if they were heavily dependent upon root vegetables in the fall, the desire for variety might push them to put in the extra effort to go hunting instead.

Fortunately and unfortunately for us, we have such incredible variety available to us that we satiate this hunger with changes not only every week, every day, and every meal but also even on every plate.

One of the challenges this creates is that the more variety we get, the more indifferent we become to variety and, therefore, the more variety we need. Where our ancestors started craving new foods after days or even weeks on the same food, we crave different foods every day and even at a single meal.

Two strategies for dealing better with variety are:

1. Letting it go for a while, focusing on a small range of tastes or foods for a period of time to reset the definition of variety. If you eat, for instance, mono-meals (meals with only one primary ingredient), you might find that your digestion is improved and that your craving for variety is reduced.

2. Learn to become creative about preparing healthy foods. (We've provided some recipes for you so you can satisfy your desire for variety without resorting to dysfunctional foods.)

A Hunger of Privilege

Recently Eric was passing through an airport when he encountered a healthy-looking organic, farm-to-table café. He ordered something to eat, and the server explained this sauce and that sauce, and in that moment, standing in an airport where he could travel, literally, anywhere in the world just by walking down a jetway, he thought about how incredibly privileged he was to be a person who could choose food based on flavor.

Think about that. Many people in the world do not have much choice about flavor, or none at all. They don't have the luxury of choosing what they eat based on how it will taste. They choose the food they need to survive. They eat what's available, when it's available, because they need it. Many of us in the Western world get to choose food based on how it tastes or because it makes us feel a certain way. The food industry has caught on to this, and they use our taste buds and our emotions against us for profit.

The fourth hunger isn't like the other hungers. It's a feeling—literally the feeling of having an **empty stomach**. Unfortunately, because most people in the Western world are always slightly malnourished, always missing certain key nutrients, they are always slightly hungry. When we feel this hunger and our stomach is empty, those feelings become linked. Very often, when we have an empty stomach, we simply feel a need to fill it.

In its natural state—say if you hadn't eaten for a few hours—your stomach should be about the size of your clenched fist. If you make a fist right now, you can get a sense of how much food you can comfortably fit into your stomach without stretching it. It's a small sack designed for the amount of food you could eat in a small period of time—food that typically required a lot of work to obtain. But our stomachs are also designed to expand. If you were part of a successful hunt, you needed to eat as much meat as you could because there was no refrigerator for leftovers. Equally, in the late summer and early fall, fruit, berries, and root veggies would be abundant, and our ancestors needed to eat as much as they could. Winter was coming, and they could not afford to miss out on the readily available calories, vitamins, and minerals.

Yet anyone who has been on a multiday fast knows that the desire to eat food largely fades away after two, three, or four days because an empty stomach isn't actually a hunger at all, it's simply a feeling that we've associated with being low on nutrients or having low blood sugar.

This week, because you are adding in all these beautiful healthy foods and maintaining your old style of eating too, it's unlikely you will experience an empty stomach feeling. As an optional upgrade to this program, you may want to experiment with a simple form of intermittent fasting: stop eating four hours before you go to bed. Even if you do this four or five days of the week, you will almost certainly experience benefits, including better sleep, more energy, and reduced cravings.

The fifth hunger is **low blood sugar**, another feeling. We have different energy sources in our body, principally sugar, fat, and, under stress, protein. For purposes of thinking about this hunger, we'll focus on sugar and fat.

Think of fat as a slow-burning, long-lasting energy source and sugar as a fast-burning, short-term energy source. Sugar is an excellent fuel for activities that take place at a moment's notice, such as sprinting. Fat is great for long-term exercise like distance running and for generally keeping your body functioning at a consistent rate. The trouble is that most people in the Western world have conditioned their bodies, through stressful lifestyles and sugar-rich diets, to burn primarily sugar.

The human body holds about 2,000 calories of blood sugar at any given time. Once that blood sugar is burned up, we enter a low blood sugar state, which produces diminished energy and, in some people, moodiness or aggressiveness. You may have heard of marathon runners who "hit the wall" around mile 17 of a 26-mile race. They stop. They simply cannot take another step because they have exhausted their available blood sugar. The body says, "We cannot burn what we do not have," and they don't finish the race.

When you are able to shift your body toward burning fat, the body relearns to generate sugar from available fat supplies on a more consistent, regular basis. What does that mean? We know one runner who completed nine marathons in seven days in the Sahara desert. It's fair to say he didn't do that burning sugar. He did it burning fat; after all, the average person carries 200,000 calories of fat with them at any given time. When your body is trained to burn fat rather than sugar, your energy becomes significantly more consistent. This is a major reason this program you have embarked on is going to be so effective for you, and so long-lasting.

The final hunger is not a hunger. It is an emotional state. We call it **emotional hunger**. Much of the food people eat is not for nutritional reasons but, rather, to change the way they feel. This is called "emotional eating" and has become an even more serious problem since the COVID-19 pandemic. People were facing tremendous personal and financial stress and often turned to food to feel better about life.

Emotional hunger sneaks up on you as an unconscious hunger that you feel can be satisfied with a particular food or type of food. We saw a great example of this with a WILDFIT client, who, at the end of the program, told Eric, "You know, my cravings are gone. My hunger is under control. For the first time in 20 years, I am looking forward to going to the beach in a two-piece bathing suit." She had experienced a major breakthrough—except for one thing.

Cake icing.

Every now and then, she had a craving for cake icing. Eric suggested that perhaps the icing reminded her of making icing with her mom, when they baked together when she was a little girl.

"No," she said. "My mom used canned icing." Then she told a story of how when she heard her mother using a can opener to open the icing can she would sneak under the table, then reach up with a spoon and blindly fish around for the can. She'd get a couple of spoonfuls before her mom caught her, after which they would laugh together.

So Eric asked her what is going on now with her mom.

She began to cry. Her mother was in early-stage dementia. At that moment she realized what she did not have to be told: her hunger for icing was a hunger to be closer to her mother, before she was sick and disappearing before her eyes.

Emotional hunger is incredibly powerful, particularly when it taps into feelings of nostalgia, a connection to the fond feelings of our past.

> *Eric: I went back to the town where I grew up—Halifax, Nova Scotia—and as I was driving, I saw a Tim Horton's, a very popular chain in Canada (imagine crossing Starbucks with Krispy Kreme). Whenever I return to Canada, I see them, but they don't mean a thing to me after 30 years of living the way we describe in this book. I'm not interested in eating there.*
>
> *But this one time, in Halifax, I was driving down the street I used to walk as a boy. I grew up going to that Tim Horton's. I went there after sporting events and for birthday parties, for all kinds of events.*
>
> *As I sat at that red light, my Food Devil said to me, "Hey, Eric, they have honey crullers in that Tim Horton's," and I literally burst out laughing. I was laughing that my Food Devil*

would even try. I have zero interest—but the fact that the idea came up, even for me, shows what an incredibly powerful force emotional hunger, and nostalgia, can be.

The way to deal with emotional hunger is to go back to the Food Timeline. Your Food Devil brings up a food that feeds an emotional hunger and says, "Hey, look at that—should we have some? Should we try it? Just one piece?" When that happens, ask yourself, "How am I feeling right now?" More importantly, ask yourself, "How do I think I'll feel after I eat that food?" Very often when the Food Devil appears, you are experiencing some sort of unpleasant emotion, perhaps loneliness or disconnection. In that moment, the Food Devil suggests that a piece of chocolate or a bowl of ice cream might stimulate you and take away the feelings of loneliness and disconnection.

The worst part is that the Food Devil isn't wrong. Eating that food might stimulate you—for a few moments at least. Just long enough for you to decide you *could* eat it. It might take the feeling away for half an hour or 45 minutes. But then you'll actually feel worse, because of the sugar rush, or the digestive problems, or the heaviness, or negative self-talk you feel.

Emotional hunger drives so many of our eating decisions. By becoming incredibly conscious, by thinking back at the food dialogue you paid attention to during Week 1 and understanding what's driving your food decisions—you'll have the powerful key for creating lasting change.

Take a Look Back

Look at what we've achieved so far. In Week 1 we asked you to drink more water. Drinking more water eliminates thirst as a hunger. Now one of your six hungers is no longer voting for bad food.

Then we asked you to breathe consciously. That creates a sense of calm. Our ancestors took the time to stop and breathe deeply only when the environment was safe. When the environment is not safe, we take rapid, shallow breaths, constantly creating cortisol and stress. If we take a moment and breathe, we calm down, and the emotional hunger has less power over us.

This week we increased the quantity of fruits, vegetables, and meats that you eat. This means you're not likely to experience any low blood sugar hunger, and the nutrition in those foods reduces your nutritional hunger. Nor will you have empty stomach hunger this week, because we are simply adding foods, and new foods address your hunger for variety.

The only hunger left to wrestle with is emotional hunger. Watch it carefully this week. If you really want to make this week work, here's what's important: Add in the things we're asking you to add in, and do not subtract things you normally would have eaten. Eat the way you normally would, and you will get to experience exactly what it's like to eat those familiar foods when all your other hungers are diminished.

You might find that your traditional foods are not as pleasurable as you thought they were. They might even cause you more discomfort than you previously realized.

1. Celebration: You are one-third of the way through the program and perhaps you have started to notice your internal food dialogue. This is a powerful step toward food freedom. Pay attention to your increased awareness and give yourself a smile or a pat on the back when you do.

2. Note from the Doctor: As the different types of hungers get quiet and you start eating more real foods (perhaps you also are eating fewer processed foods), is your fasting blood glucose level starting to change for the better? Watch your fasting glucose closely and be compulsive about testing and logging it. Make an appointment with your health provider to let him or her know that you want them along for your journey.

   The medical profession is changing, becoming more accepting of nonpharmacologic modalities of glucose control (nondrug treatments). I want

to tell you a doctor's secret. We doctors have all
the same diseases that you do, including diabetes,
hypertension, and bad lipids. We too get fatty liver,
retinopathy leading to blindness, kidney failure
leading to dialysis, poor circulation leading to
amputations, heart attacks, and strokes. We really do
know that lifestyle measures, including diet, exercise,
sleep, stress reduction, and loving and supportive
relationships all affect our glucose. We just don't
know how to inspire or teach. We have minimal time
with patients to educate them and very little training
on effective methodologies to share with them. In
regard to diet lifestyle, we don't have a clue about
effective methodologies to recommend. I'm hoping
that you become an ambassador to my profession
by getting your provider involved in your journey
and give us hope that there is truly a way to affect
lifestyle change.

3. Tips for Success

    – Remove nothing (continue to eat normally),
      increase fruits and veggies, keep up your water
      intake, do the breathing exercises, and pay
      attention to your food dialogue and the Food
      Timeline while also observing which of the Six
      Human Hungers you might experience.

    – To make this work, add things in; don't
      subtract anything.

    – Review the summary of what we've achieved in
      Weeks 1 and 2.

    – Pay attention, drink water, breathe, and bring in
      more fruits and vegetables.

    – There is only one hunger left: emotional; watch
      it carefully and think about alternative ways of
      neutralizing it.

WEEK 3

Welcome to Week 3 and congratulations for completing Week 2! As we come to the end of Phase I (the first three weeks), this week we're going to make one change, and it's a big one. It's going to have a significant impact on your eating decisions, because we are going to take a break this week from all added sugars.

What does this mean? It means cane sugar. It means corn syrup. It means sugar under all the various names the food industry uses to hide sugar. (Last time we counted, we came up with 65 terms used to describe and hide sugar on labels.¶) We're going to be free from sugar in all the obvious ways, and all the non-obvious ways, which means it will be important for you to read nutritional labels.

There are two different parts to these labels. One is the ingredients, and the other is the nutritional constituents. If you look at the nutritional breakdown, you will see there is sugar in all kinds of things, and that's fine—the nutritional breakdown on an apple, for instance, will show sugar. What we're interested in is when sugar shows up on the *ingredients* list. That's added sugar. This week we are going to be free from that kind of sugar, and it might be challenging because you are about to find out, if you were not already aware, that that sugar is in just about *everything*.

Remember what we learned about the sugar industry? Now is the time to see the sugar industry as drug dealers; they put sugar in everything to take away your freedom. As we described in Chapter 2, sugar has been added to your food very intentionally by the food industry. They intend to stimulate your appetite and make you hungrier so you'll eat more than you need to and they can enjoy increased profits.

This may be disheartening. You may think, *What am I going to eat?* But don't worry. We've developed a variety of delicious recipes to help you at this stage.**

¶   Learn more at www.PostDiabetes.com/links/65NamesofSugar.

**   Visit www.PostDiabetes.com/links/Week3Recipes to view the recipes.

It probably doesn't surprise you to know that sugar is the second or third most common ingredient in most breakfast cereals (there are exceptions to this—sugar should be the *first* ingredient in Lucky Charms, but they have managed to keep it at number two by listing corn syrup and dextrose separately down the list.)

What may surprise you is to discover how prevalent sugar is in foods where you wouldn't expect it.

> *Eric: When I took my first sugar holiday many years ago, I ran home one day to make a quick, sugar-free lunch. I boiled some pasta and grabbed a jar of what I believed to be a fairly healthy organic pasta sauce. I'd been without sugar for a full week and was pleased with how things were going.*
>
> *I poured the sauce over the pasta, took a bite—and literally spat it back onto the plate. I was convinced that the sauce in the jar must have gone bad.*
>
> *I checked the expiry date, and it was fine. I tried another small taste and realized that it tasted like candy.*
>
> *What I hadn't quite realized is that, during the sugar-free week, my taste buds had been adjusting to their new environment. If your taste buds are constantly slammed by refined sugar, corn syrup, artificial sweeteners, and so on, they become a bit deadened to sweetness. They need to experience more and more sweetness just to register it and to satisfy that craving.*

What Eric experienced when he took a bite of pasta sauce was a blast of added sugar—it was the number two ingredient in his supposedly healthy pasta, more common even than tomatoes. The sauce hadn't gone bad at all; it was just so sweet to his adjusted taste buds that it seemed to be off.

Sugar is added to everything.

This week you may find yourself disappointed. You may read the label on a food you like to eat and notice that it has added sugar. Disappointment seems like a natural response—but don't give into it.

Instead of feeling disappointed, feel angry.

Disappointment will lead you to eat that food. The Food Devil will use disappointment to pry open the door and convince you that eating the food will make you feel better, the way eating used to make you feel better. "Look," the Food Devil will tell you, "it's not that much. Sugar is in everything anyway. You may as well eat it; you can't fight it. Anyway, who wants the hassle of eating something else?"

The sugar is there to get you to buy and eat more food than you need. The sugar is there to boost profitability for companies that don't care about your health. The sugar in that food is one of the reasons you are in the condition that has you reading this book right now.

Instead of feeling disappointed by the realization that your favorite foods contain unnecessary added sugar, feel angry. Very angry. The sugar is there to hook you and boost their profits at the cost of your health and quality of life.

Feel angry enough to smash that food on the floor. Okay, you probably shouldn't actually smash it—but do put it back on the shelf. Don't buy it. Go find the store manager and say, "Why is there added sugar in every single tomato sauce you sell?" If enough of us do this over time, you will not only have a massive impact on your own health but also on food manufacturing around the world.

1. Celebration: Each time you resist sugar, celebrate. Every time you discover sugar somewhere that surprises you, celebrate. This is an important week; for many it will be the beginning of freedom from sugar.

2. Note from the Doctor: Wow, removing processed sugar will have a major effect on your blood glucose levels! Processed dietary sugars enter your blood system at lightning speed and cause massive glucose spikes and insulin responses. Sugars from fruit and vegetables have far less sugar in comparison and take much more time to digest. Far less insulin is needed, and there is markedly less glucose in the bloodstream.

Be extra careful now, especially if you're taking medications that stay in your system a long time. Sulfonylureas (for example, glipizide or glyburide) and meglitinides (for example, repaglinide) should be stopped. These medications stay in your body a long time and can cause hypoglycemia or low blood glucose for days. Get your medical provider on board. Find out if you're on one of these types of medications. Tell your provider that you're on a low-carbohydrate diet and get him or her excited. Check your glucose daily. Consider reducing your insulin by half as your fasting and after-meal glucose levels come down. Watch closely for symptoms of hypoglycemia, including tremor, palpitations, anxiety/arousal, sweating, pallor, hunger, paresthesia, dizziness, weakness, drowsiness, and confusion or altered mental status. Let your doctor know right away if you're experiencing any symptoms.

3.   Tips for Success

   –   Continue to build on the progress from Weeks 1 and 2 and take a holiday from added sugar.

   –   Willpower *does* work, but only for short bursts of effort. Diets fail people because they ask people to *rely* on willpower to change their habits; we are asking you to *use* willpower for a short time in order to create long-term freedom for you. This does not mean that you will never eat sugar again; it means that you will only do so consciously.

CHAPTER 5

Phase II: WILDFIT Spring

As we begin the second phase of this project, let's recap what we've done so far.

In Week 1, we took a look at food psychology. You discovered that you have a lot of personalities when it comes to food. Then you learned about your food dialogue and the Six Human Hungers. By now you have an increased consciousness about the way you make food decisions.

You may have found that increased consciousness has begun to have a positive impact on your food decisions. You may be finding it easier to say no to things you used to want, and harder to say yes. This is a sign that you are headed toward real food freedom.

When we moved into Week 2, we worked on one of the most important principles of nutrition: your health is determined far more by getting the good stuff than by not eating bad stuff. We worked on increasing the quantity and quality of the healthy foods you are taking in but didn't ask you to cut back on anything you are accustomed to eating.

In Week 3 we made one change: cut out added sugar in all its many guises. We asked you to pay attention to where sugar is found in your diet. We also asked you to pay attention to the way you respond when you learn there is sugar in foods you'd like to eat. You could react with a sense of disappointment, which triggers an inner temper tantrum and may even cause you to eat that food you know has sugar in it. Or you could remember why that sugar is there—that it is an ingredient inserted by the food industry in order to manipulate you—and react with indignation or anger. That reaction can empower you to put that food down and move on.

And remember, the best way for us to change the food industry is to change ourselves; when we stop buying things, they stop making them.

SEASONAL EATING

As we enter the second phase, you are probably starting to have a different view of yourself, your relationship with food, and the food industry. Phase II respects the fact that our ancestors evolved to live through a variety of seasons. When we say "seasons," remember we're not talking about the Northern Hemisphere. We're not talking about the kind of winters people experience in Minnesota or the summers of Eastern Europe. We're talking about seasons in sub-Saharan Africa where our species originated and evolved.

As the human body evolved, it did so in response to the natural environment that our ancestors lived in. As the seasons in Africa changed, food availability changed, and our bodies evolved to survive and where possible thrive through these seasons.

For instance, in one season—say late summer or fall—there may have been an abundance of berries or root vegetables. During this season, the pancreas would devote energy to the production of insulin, which would break down sugars for immediate use and longer-term energy storage as glycogen or fat.

As the seasons shifted, the body's functions would shift also, adapting to survive the new conditions presented by the new season. Moving out of fall and into winter, the pancreas—as we discussed in Chapter 2—moves from producing insulin to producing glucagon so that the body can switch fuel sources and burn stored fat.

The pancreas does not produce these hormones (insulin and glucagon) at the same time. It does one job at a time. One of the challenges that comes about as a result of modern humans no longer eating in seasonal patterns is that we fall victim to a use-it-or-lose-it situation. If your pancreas is only asked to do one job—make insulin—then you may strain it doing that job, and at the same time let its ability to do the other job atrophy. Your pancreas wants you to go through the seasons for which it evolved. Mother Nature used to force those seasons upon you; now you must use some willpower to make sure you live in a way that is optimal for your body.

Our bodies evolved to optimize function for and to survive each of the seasons and the transitions between the seasons. For instance, the body "knows" that winter follows fall and learned, therefore, to use the carb-rich fall season to fatten up for the winter season. Some of those seasons had a great abundance of certain kinds of foods. Some were abundant in other foods. And some seasons lacked food entirely. Our ancestors evolved the ability to survive this variability. But starvation was very real and a significant cause of death. Food was not something you got by walking into a building and handing over a piece of plastic. Acquiring food might involve going on an incredibly long hunting trip or scouring the countryside, looking for seasonal berries or tubers. The job of hunting and gathering required a huge amount of effort and was always unpredictable. As a result, our ancestors were often on the doorstep of starvation. We've evolved some interesting physiology to deal with that. One of the capabilities we developed was the ability to store energy in fat. Fat is a reliable source of hydration and energy.

Here is one way to look at energy/fat storage.

When one of our ancestors encountered an abundance of carbohydrate-rich foods (fruit, root vegetables, tubers, honey), their bodies evolved a complex energy-saving system that works a bit like money. Think of blood sugar as, say, money in your wallet. When you consume carbs, your body has to decide what to do with it. The first thing it will do is make sure that you have enough energy for right now, and it does this by topping up your blood sugar—making sure that your wallet is full of spending cash.

Once your wallet is full—that is, your blood sugar is at maximum—your body will take the surplus sugars and put them into a savings account. For the sake of our metaphor, that savings account is glycogen stored in your liver and in your muscles.

Once your liver and muscles are full of glycogen, your body will then make "term deposits" for long-term savings; it will store the surplus energy as fat.

And so when you eat carb-rich foods in excess of your energy requirements, you are more likely to store fat and make it hard to release fat.

When a winter drought occurs, plants become scarce and animal populations dwindle. Hunting becomes more difficult. Food is generally harder to come by. But that was okay if you were a Paleolithic man or woman, because your body knew this season was coming. In the same way that a squirrel stores nuts in preparation for winter, your body stored energy in fat for the African winter: the dry season. This increased your chances of survival and passing on your genetic material. And so, humans have become incredibly good at processing seasonal carbs and surviving long periods without carbs at all.

The challenge today is we don't face any seasonal fluctuation or rotation from a nutritional perspective. You may live in a place that has a long, snowy winter, but that has no impact on your available food supply. You can go to the store and buy bananas year-round. You can buy oranges or meat whenever you want. As far as food is concerned, you do not face seasonality any longer.

This creates a number of challenges. One is that you can cause malnutrition by eating foods you prefer over the foods you would have been forced to eat because there was nothing else. Before agriculture, shops, restaurants, and food delivery, seasonal rotation forced healthy nutritional variety.

Further, this lack of seasonal rotation means your body might get stuck in one mode—say, "saving for winter" mode—and, as a result, create a series of imbalances or injuries with health implications.

Phase II will gently introduce you to what we call Spring mode, which will help your body achieve ketosis; your body will produce ketones, and you will switch to burning fat as your primary fuel source and recalibrate your insulin sensitivity.

We are going to achieve this by building upon what we have done so far and then doing some things that will "trick" the body into believing that it is sub-Saharan spring so that your body can go into Spring mode and start correcting some of the imbalances you are experiencing by living a "modern" lifestyle.

So, as we move into Week 4, let's begin some internal "spring cleaning."

WEEK 4

Welcome to Week 4, when spring is in the air. Okay—spring may not *actually* be in the air where you are when you read this, but it is metaphorically in the air for you, because we are going to make two lifestyle changes atop the foundation we have built in the past three weeks that will create fabulous changes in your body.

This week we'll show you how to shift your pancreas from producing insulin to producing glucagon so you can begin burning fat. We promise we won't let you get hungry! And we'll invite you to try out two optional experiments that might just take your health to an entirely new level.

Fat-Burning Mode

Spring is a fascinating season in sub-Saharan Africa, the place of our species origin and where most of our evolution took place. Amazing things happen in spring. Antelopes like gazelles, for instance, have a multiweek breeding cycle, yet they all have their babies pretty much on the same day in spring—the day of the first rains. They evolved this behavior as a defense against hungry predators who survived the winter. If the antelope herd were to drop a few babies on Monday and a few babies on Tuesday and a few babies on Wednesday, the lions and hyenas and wild dogs and leopards and Paleolithic humans would hunt and eat them all. But by birthing them all on the same day, using the rain as a catalyst, they give their babies a fighting chance. The carnivores can only eat so much on that day, and this gives the baby antelopes who survive the first few days of life time to find their legs and get up to speed.

In addition to the abundance of meat during the rain, there is also an immediate increase in greens. Spring for us, then, is a low-glycemic season, focused on eating high-quality lean proteins and a wide variety of fresh and new vegetables.

By mimicking, to some degree, the way our ancestors ate in their spring, we can "tell" our bodies to move into Spring mode and start correcting the imbalances we have discussed.

As we mentioned at the end of the last chapter, this means that your body will start burning fat, or ketones, rather than sugar, or carbohydrates, as your primary energy source. Last week we removed added sugars from your diet, particularly the dangerous ones you might never want to go back to, like refined sugars, corn syrup, and so on. This week we're going to take a break from all sugars, including those that are not so obviously harmful. We're going to take a break from grains like wheat, rice, quinoa, and corn. We're going to take a break from staple foods that you may have gotten used to, like bread and pasta. We're going to take a break from root vegetables like sweet potatoes, yams, and carrots. We're going to take a break from honey. In fact, this week we are going to take a break from all carbohydrate-rich foods.

If you are vegetarian, vegan, or would simply prefer to avoid animal products, we have created a video and guidebook to support you through Gatherer's Spring, a version of Spring that does not involve meat, fish, eggs, or other animal products.

Alternatively, if you are sensitive to many vegetables or if you are dealing with excessive inflammation, you might want to try Hunter's Spring, a version of Spring that is more carnivore focused or meat based. On our website, we have provided a video and guidebook to support you with Hunter's Spring if you prefer that option.

The key, whichever version of Spring you choose, is to take a break from carbohydrate-rich foods. Of course, it may not be possible to avoid all carbohydrates, but the keys are to avoid all junk carbs and to keep your carb intake below 25 grams per day; the *deeper* you want to go into Spring, the lower that number should be.

But remember, we are only taking a break. For a season. To achieve specific things.

By taking this break, you will push your body into fat-burning mode. Your pancreas will ease up on producing insulin, necessary to process and store carbohydrates as glycogen and fat, and switch to making glucagon, to burn stored fat. At the same time, we are going to step up the amount of exercise we get—not tremendously, but noticeably. We're not asking you to suddenly take up yoga or start going to the gym. What we are asking you to do is consider your regular exercise routine and add to it something we call "intentional movement."

We Were Born to Move

Our ancestors lived in an environment where not moving wasn't an option. If they didn't move, they would die. On a recent hunting trip with the Hadza bushmen, I [Eric] carried a GPS tracker so I could see precisely where and how far the group went in its daily hunting and gathering. I have run a marathon, and I can tell you this was five times as hard, because we were going up and down steep hills and pushing through thorn bushes. One day we walked, jogged, and ran 27 miles (43 km) in temperatures up to 107°F (42°C). And, although we covered a lot of ground, we came back empty-handed.

The very next day, the chief, who I know well, came up to me and asked, in a teasing way, "Do you want to go again?" Physical exertion is an everyday activity for the Hadza, much as it must have been for our ancestors. After a 27-mile marathon, they were going out to hunt again. That second day we went 18 miles (29 km), and our venture was more successful: we found a lot of plant foods and got a huge bush pig.

If the Hadza had not gone out again that morning, we would not have eaten. Today, most of us have lives in which we face a tremendous variety and quantity of available foods. We can eat simply by pushing a button.

We don't move nearly as much as our bodies were designed to, mostly because we don't have to. In fact, I have watched the Hadza; they don't move any more than they have to. They are very good energy conservationists, but nature forces them to move.

It is also important to realize that as well as being good for energy use, metabolism, muscle growth, and bone density, there is another very important reason to move.

Your lymphatic system is a network of tissues and organs that help cleanse the body of toxins, waste, and other unwanted materials. Crucially, it does not have a pump.

Because blood flow is both urgent and important, we have a heart. Oxygen, too, is both urgent and important, and so we have a diaphragm. These pumps make sure that our bodies' urgent needs are taken care of.

Lymphatic flow is important but not urgent in the same way as oxygen is, so our bodies evolved a different way without creating another pump. Our bodies simply use our normal day-to-day movements and resulting muscle contractions to move lymph around.

But what do you think happens when we don't move enough? Not enough lymph flow, not enough cleansing, and a resulting buildup of toxins, waste, and other unwanted materials.

This week, we are going to talk about how to keep your body moving without having to do any crazy exercise.

Start to Move

This week, all we are going to ask you to do is think about your normal patterns of movement. If you're quite sedentary, then we are going to ask you to start moving a bit. If you're already active, we are only asking you to increase your aerobic output. We're not asking you to lift more when you are at the gym, or even go to the gym if you didn't before. We just want you to start looking for opportunities to move a bit more and take a few extra steps.

Examples of doing a little bit more might include giving up the rock-star parking spot at work, parking on the far edge of the lot, and walking to the front door. Or instead of always taking the elevator, make a decision that this week, if you're going three or fewer floors, you'll skip the elevator (and the escalator) and take the stairs. If you're in an airport, skip the moving sidewalks. Find a way to increase your step count. (Here's the great news: Every one of us carries a pedometer. Smart phones today either have step counters built in, or you can download an app to do that. This will allow you to track how many steps you take each day and actively work to increase that number.)

Don't Get Hungry

It is important, this week and moving forward, that you don't let yourself get hungry. When spring arrived for our ancestors, it was a magical time. Imagine what it would have been like to go for weeks or months without a ready supply of water or food. Then, at last, you see dark clouds forming on the horizon of the savanna. In the evening you catch the distant flash of flickering lightning. A sense of hope builds up in your chest, for you know the rains are coming. As the rains begin to fall, all the animals begin giving birth, for they know that the grasses are about to reappear. In the coming days, green shoots sprout up everywhere, changing the hue of the landscape overnight.

In just a few days, you have moved from a time of scarcity to a time of abundance. During this week, we want you to simulate that as best you can. Increase your intake of bitter, healthy leafy greens and other vegetables. Increase your intake of healthy proteins (if you're a vegetarian, this may be more difficult but could involve eating more nuts, legumes, or lentils or, if you're a flexitarian, eggs and fish). If you're not a vegetarian, look for the best-quality, ethically raised, healthiest protein sources you can get. Examples include bison, free-range organic beef, wild-caught fish, or free-range poultry. If these versions are unavailable or out of your reach, then just get the best quality you can.

The important thing is, even as you avoid carbohydrates this week, don't let yourself go hungry at all. (Remember, if you feel hungry, eat within the season, and if you don't feel like eating any of the in-season foods, then you probably aren't actually hungry and may want to remind yourself of the Six Human Hungers to see what is making you want to eat.)

This will be a change for your body. It is going to need to catch up. Your gut microbiome will alter and adjust as you move into a new season, so your digestion might be a bit off for a few days. You may, at first, find yourself struggling for energy as your body reluctantly gives up its sugar diet and slowly moves toward living on fat. For some people this transition is quick, like flipping a switch. Others find it takes days and days and feels more like a slow dimmer switch.

If you find yourself struggling with very low energy, don't give in to the craving that is pushing you toward a nonfunctional carbohydrate or sugary food. Instead, during the first few days, have a little fresh fruit on an empty stomach or a few root veggies. On day one, eat a little bit in the morning. On day two, a little bit less. Day three, even less. The goal is to be free of even those carbs by day four so you can truly enter Spring.

Stick to it. You might find yourself developing a rash or feel like you are developing a cold or the flu. These things are a normal part of switching to spring for the first time in many years. You will get through to the other side and will feel fantastic.

Break Time

Also during Week 4, we invite you to take a break from three interesting substances that you might very well not want to leave behind right away. We're asking you to think about this week by week.

The first of those substances is alcohol.

Pay attention here—did you just react to that statement with anger? Fear? Or perhaps curiosity? Did you think, *I'm not sure I can do that?* The more emotional your response to that statement was, the more valuable this break is going to be for you.

The key thing to understand is that in order to trigger Spring in the body, we have to move away from carbs, and alcohol is a significant carbohydrate injection into your system. So for this week you're going to take a complete break from alcohol.

The second substance we're going to step away from for a while may be a tad controversial—when Eric chose to walk away from it 20 years ago, people thought he was downright crazy. That's because 20 years ago, dairy products—your other break candidate—were considered essential. They were considered a necessary feature of the human diet. We were told that if we didn't consume dairy products, our bones would be weak and we would suffer other health repercussions.

We are aware now that this is not the case.[1] We know that message was the product of marketing manipulation and lobbying. We are aware that mammals should probably only be drinking milk that came from their own species and should stop when they develop their teeth. (Other than humans, no adult mammals in the world continue drinking milk.) We know that dairy products are not required for human health. And so we're suggesting that you take a holiday from dairy products—from milk and cheese and cream and yogurt. Don't worry, it's just a break for now. (Grass-raised butter or ghee are a notable exception.)

The third substance to take a break from this week is processed oils, including vegetable or seed oils. Do what you can to reduce or avoid them by choosing olive oil, coconut oil, or ghee in their stead.

Even More Breaks!

There are two more breaks we would like to recommend, but you should only take these steps if you feel inspired to. We ask you to stick to the other changes we have recommended, but these two are optional.

What we've told you up to now is about creating the WILD-FIT Spring state of ketosis in your body. These other two are worth stepping away from in order to improve your overall health, period. They will support your body's healing efforts.

The first is caffeine.

If you're having a big, emotional reaction to that, it's a clue for you. It means now is definitely time for a break. If you're driving late at night, it's 3 A.M. and you're tired, then caffeine is a great idea. Caffeine can help you maintain awareness and get through that long drive. But when your caffeine use crosses over to the point where you cannot function, where you cannot be human, where you cannot be friendly to the people around you without it, then you've given up your freedom. You've been imprisoned by caffeine.

This week we ask you to break out of that prison. Take a break from caffeine and experience what it's like not to be controlled by a substance that is, remember, a plant-produced insecticide that stimulates your adrenal glands, keeping you awake or making it more difficult for you to drop into the healthy, natural sleep that your body requires.

Caffeine pumps cortisol and epinephrine (adrenaline) into your system; this is why it *feels* nice. Caffeine doesn't simply stop you from sleeping. It also damages the quality of your sleep.

Quitting caffeine might seem hard, but we have good news for you. We have worked with thousands of people from over 100 countries around the world. Many of our clients have told us that taking a break from caffeine right here, right now, after the changes you've made so far, has reduced their withdrawal symptoms. Previously they might have faced monstrous headaches that would cause tremendous suffering and interrupt their personal and professional lives. When they stop caffeine at this point in the program, on the other hand, they may have experienced only a distant, foggy headache that lasted for a few hours or a day. In some cases, people experienced no withdrawal at all.

Taking a break from caffeine now could be a remarkable gift to your body. This could be the opportunity you've been waiting for to lessen that dependency you sometimes feel. Imagine the benefits: lowered blood pressure, deeper sleep, an uplifted mood, decreased anxiety, fewer midnight bathroom visits, healthier gums and teeth, reduced risk of cardiac events, and naturally, saving money.

This could be the perfect moment for you to discover a newfound freedom from caffeine. And with that freedom, envision the joy of savoring caffeinated drinks, and their effects, more consciously in the future.

This is an optional step in the program, but we hope you will at least give it a try; if you do and you can't stick with it, no worries. Just stick with the rest of the program.

The next substance we invite you to take an optional break from, if you use it, is tobacco, for many of the same reasons. There's plenty of information about why you should stop using tobacco—we're not going to rehash that here, but you might want to watch this video* about nicotine addiction that will give you a perspective that you may not have considered before. You know the reasons. Instead of giving you reasons, we're going to give you good news.

The good news is that, as with caffeine, our clients have reported that this was the easiest possible time for them to give up tobacco. Instead of worrying about quitting, stressing about quitting, or trying to quit for weeks on end, they found that after a few days of no tobacco, the voices inside demanding it calmed down and in a few weeks were gone entirely. The withdrawal symptoms that used to plague them when they tried to quit before simply vanished and, because they were in Spring when they did it, they didn't end up with the usual weight gain that comes along with trying to quit smoking.

This moment might just be the right time to radically change your relationship not only with food—which you are already doing—and with caffeine, but also with tobacco.

1. Celebration: Are you gaining any feelings of freedom about food? You have completed three weeks and laid an excellent foundation to move into an incredibly

---

* Visit www.PostDiabetes.com/links/nicotineaddiction to learn more.

important step in your recovery: Spring. How much stronger do you feel about your food choices? Which cravings are getting weaker? Where are you feeling better?

2. Note from the Doctor: This is the week where super-dramatic changes in your glucose occur. It is critical to follow your glucose closely. Consider increasing your testing to three times daily: first thing in the morning, before dinner, and at bedtime. Ask your health provider if you can check in daily. Remember the sulfonylureas and meglitinides? They stay in the body a long time, and your provider will definitely stop those medications or adjust your insulin dosage, and they might just stop all diabetic medications completely. I would if you were my patient! Let your provider know that you are entering a very low-carbohydrate week or weeks. Have him or her review hypoglycemic symptoms with you. Your body's conversion to a fat-burning metabolism might take a few days, since it still has access to simple glucose in the form of glycogen stored in your liver and muscles. If you have a blood pressure cuff, take your blood pressure two to three times daily. You might be able to stop or reduce your blood pressure medications too.

3. Tips for Success

   – This week, we are going to build on the progress and move into Spring mode by taking a break from all remaining carbohydrates and focusing on low-sugar vegetables, Alkagizer smoothies, good-quality proteins with healthy fats, and intentional movement. Remember from the first three weeks: stay hydrated, do some breathing exercises every day, and pay close attention to your emotions and internal dialogue. And do not let yourself get hungry.

- Sometimes when people go on diets, they think a little cheat is okay as long as it is small or as long as they do some exercise to work it off. That is a broken paradigm; every single day that you tell your body that it is Spring will move you toward recovery and energy. A slight "cheat" with carbs tells your body that perhaps winter is on the way back and will push your pancreas into "winter is coming" mode, which is the last thing you want right now. If you do experiment with any carbs, learn from it and move on. Your goal here is as many days in a row in Spring; this is not the week for experimenting with carbs.

WEEK 5

Welcome to Week 5! Before you continue—are you reading ahead? Because if you are, we really do mean it when we ask you to put the book down and allow yourself to thrive through Week 4 properly.

Still reading? Then congratulations on completing Week 4 and the first four weeks of your transformation. As we move into Week 5, we're going to remain in Spring. There are no real changes for you to make at this point, but there are some things for you to be aware of. Continue what you've been doing. Remind yourself of why you're doing it. And begin to build a tribe that supports you.

You may encounter some speed bumps this week, but we want you to see them as progress that your body is doing the right things to support your transformation. You may also, for instance, have low energy for a time while your body makes the switch from burning sugar to burning fat. You may also develop some rashes or itchy skin, and it is even possible that you develop some cold or flu-like symptoms. While these things might be unpleasant, they are a normal part of correcting the imbalance that you are so close to remedying. This is a great time to reach out to an accountability partner or a coach.

Remember Your Why

If you are struggling with cravings, go back and think about all you have achieved since you began. Think about how you took a look at your own psychology and how you examined the dialogue that you have with yourself about food. The arguments between your Food Devil and your Food Angel have probably changed a lot over the past four weeks. The Food Devil may still be doing its work. If you feel bad, if your energy is down, the Food Devil may say, "What the hell is this all about? This doesn't seem to be helping at all. We're worse off than we were before. We should just go get an ice cream and an apple pie."

That's drug dealer talk. That's exactly what a drug dealer would say as you came to the end of a withdrawal period: "You can end the withdrawal. You don't have to feel sick like this. Just have another hit." Be aware that your Food Devil might do this to you this week. Stay strong.

It's important that you pay attention to two things. One, why are you doing this? Why do you want to make this change? Who do you want to be at the end of it? What kind of lifestyle do you want? Do you want to be off your medications? Do you want to stop taking injections? Do you want to have good circulation and good health, to think of yourself not as someone living with a disease but as someone who has recovered from an injury?

This might be a good time to take out your journal and reflect on your reasons. Why is this important to you? What are the benefits to you in sticking with this? What are the costs of giving in to the food industry? The more clarity you can create about why you are doing this, the easier it will be to push through any tough minutes, hours, or days.

Two, pay attention to the progress you've made so far. Look back through your journal. Have you noticed your relationship with food is a little different? Have you noticed any changes in your body? Have you noticed any changes in your psychology? The more you are able to notice these indirect wins, the more those wins will help you see that you are making progress—and progress is fundamental to motivation. When people feel a complete lack of progress, it's difficult for them to maintain motivation, so it's important to notice any indirect wins you are experiencing. And to celebrate them.

Are you having an easier time making food decisions? Is the Food Devil having a harder time winning arguments? Are you sleeping better? Does your skin look better? How about your hair? Pay attention to all these things and look for the micro wins. Those wins will keep you on track and give you energy to keep going.

We have provided you with several recipes in the back of the book that are perfect for this week and will help you stay excited about healthy food and the progress you are making.

The Monkey Lesson

In South Africa, there's a sanctuary designed for primates rescued from captivity: unwanted pets, circus animals, and so on. People who have primates as pets soon realize that they don't make good pets, and they surrender them.

The sanctuary is home to many exotic species of rescued monkeys, but they also have a healthy population of vervet monkeys, a local and endemic species. The sanctuary is surrounded by very high fences, but without an enclosure at the top, the fences could never keep the vervet monkeys in. And this worried the owners of the sanctuary at first. Because it is too big for a fully enclosed fencing system, they were worried that the vervets would leave once they start bringing in exotic monkeys.

Why would that worry them? Why would they want the vervets to stay?

The answer: to teach the other monkeys.

When new monkeys are brought to the sanctuary, they are put in quarantine cages for two to three weeks. They sit in those cages with their hands on the bars and spend all their time watching the other monkeys. When they are released into the sanctuary, they don't become pals. They don't become friends. But they do watch the vervets very, very carefully.

Why is this? Many of these primates come from other parts of Africa or even other parts of the world. They are now in a forest where they have no idea what is edible and what is not. They learn what to eat and what is toxic by observing and mimicking the behavior of vervet monkeys.

You can do the same thing.

You are now in a very important stage, because you've decided to eat slightly differently. You're now in Spring. One of the ways you can support yourself is by identifying other people who are living this way—people who are health conscious and who have decided to move away from the heavy carbohydrate diet that is damaging their bodies. Think about reaching out and connecting with people who you know are eating well; eating at restaurants that are focused on healthy food; and learning about healthy dieting and healthy lifestyles. Look for people who can really support the changes you are making right now.

Please reach out and join the Post Diabetic Facebook group where you will find like-minded people on a similar journey. You will make new friends, share restaurant and recipe tips, and help each other stay on track. As the African proverb says, "If you want to go fast, go alone. If you want to go far, go together."

Recognize, too, the value a strong social community can provide beyond the critical element of teaching. Laughter, touch, and love are an important part of a healthy lifestyle. These things may not seem related to your sugar management or your fat storage, but they are directly related. Imagine for a moment that you somehow got separated from your clan a hundred thousand years ago. You're now alone in the wilderness. Your adrenaline and cortisol levels shoot up. Wouldn't it be vital for you to be extremely good at storing fat? Because now you are on your own, and the more alone and isolated you feel, the more your body will do what it can to protect you. Overstoring fat and processing sugar badly are exactly the evolutionary result of the body's response to that kind of stress. Reduce that stress, and that response, by making sure you have strong social connections and expressions of affection. That will really help your recovery.

For many of you, this is the farthest you've gotten in a diet program, or the longest you've been able to stick with one. The Food Devil is probably starting to speak up and congratulate you, saying, "Hey, man, you should celebrate with some pizza and ice cream!" Here's what we suggest you do instead. In this video[†] we discuss the 25 common reasons people bail out of any diet program. Instead of listening to the Food Devil, watch the video. And then congratulate yourself.

1. Celebration: Well done! You have completed your first week of Spring; you are doing so well. Watch for the speed bumps (rashes, low energy, cold-like symptoms) and celebrate if they happen. They are a sign that you are on the right track.

    Notice, too, whether any of your cravings are going down. Is the Food Angel winning more easily? Are you starting to feel increased levels of food freedom?

2. Note from the Doctor: Are you amazed yet that your fasting sugar is close to normal, if not completely normal, and that you are getting more and more energy? This is the week I really started believing that I could control my life simply by putting in the good stuff and removing the bad stuff. Being the proverbial doctor who had to "heal thyself," could I really live without pills? Remember, I had started this program taking 10 different medications. By this point, I had already stopped the diabetes and cholesterol pills, and this week began to reduce my blood pressure medications. My sugars were normal and repeated BP checks confirmed that my blood pressure was the best it had been in a very long time. To say that I was amazed is an understatement!

---

† http://www.postdiabetes.com/links/whydietsfail

3. Tips for Success

    –   No enhancements this week; stay in Spring.
        Focus on eating a lot of good stuff (low-carb
        veggies, quality proteins, and fats), stay hydrated,
        do your breathing exercises, and make sure that
        you are getting some good movement in.

    –   Stick with it. When the Food Devil tries to
        convince you to celebrate your success with
        carbs, laugh and drink some water. You are
        making such excellent progress; focus on that
        and know that you are doing wonderful things
        for your body.

WEEK 6

Welcome to Week 6. Do we need to say it again? Have you completed Week 5? Please do not read on until you have!

Of course, if you have, congratulations! You're now two weeks into Spring. By now you should be feeling the benefits of this season. This week you continue in Spring, and we invite you to stretch your wings a bit.

This is an incredibly exciting time for many people. It is the first time their body has experienced Spring mode, or ketosis. This may be the first time you've given your pancreas a break from heavy insulin production and asked it to manufacture glucagon on a regular basis. This change may take some adjustment, as you may have experienced. If you are among the small minority of people still struggling for energy at this point, or still suffering from some transitional symptoms such as rashes or flu-like symptoms, don't give up. We know about 10 percent of our clients fall into this category and may even go into the third week feeling this way. But we also know things will get better for you, so hang in there.

If you would like some additional support at this stage, please remember to post in the Post Diabetic Facebook group or request a discovery call with one of our coaches.

Are You Bored?

Now that you've been in WILDFIT Spring for some weeks, you may be experiencing a bit of boredom. You're eating the same things over and over again. Think about this, though: our ancestors did not have much choice when it came to food. The food available was the food available, no matter how sick and tired they were of it. Today, we are plagued by an onslaught of variety. And 90 percent of that variety is products that are addictive, life-shortening, designed primarily for food manufacturer profitability, and absolutely not about your optimal health or quality of life.

If you feel like you're struggling a little bit this week, or you want some variety, remember that we have provided a number of recipes in the appendices and that you can swap and share recipes with others in the Facebook group.

Our next challenge for you is not to make changes of any kind. It's to stay in Spring and learn how to make Spring fun. For instance, we invite you to learn how to order in a restaurant in a way that's fun.

Now, you may be one of those people who struggles when it comes time to order in a restaurant. You don't want to be *that person* who says, "Oh, can I have this, but without that, and would you mind checking if it has added sugar?"

We want to remind you of something about *that person. That person* is statistically far less likely to get cancer. *That person* is much less likely to have long-term blood sugar management problems. *That person* is much less likely to have respiratory or heart disease. *That person* is going to live a higher quality of life because they were willing to put themselves first and not let shame hold them—*you*—back.

How to Eat Out

From now on, when you order in a restaurant, understand that every menu is simply a badly organized list of ingredients. The menu lists the ingredients the restaurant has, and that's useful to you. You can read the menu and say, "Oh, they have wild-caught salmon and linguini over here, and they have cheese-smothered broccoli over here. That means they have salmon, linguini, broccoli, and cheese." Choose the ingredients you really want, turn to the server, and say, "I'd like to have the wild-caught salmon and the broccoli, but I'm not interested in the linguini or the cheese."

The server is going to tell you there is an extra charge for that. You smile and say, "Thank you! I am happy to pay that extra charge, because it's worth it." (Think of how much it will save you in medical and drug costs.)

This week, stretch your wings. Learn how to prepare healthy snacks and make sure you keep them nearby. Learn how to cook different meals and how to order in a restaurant with a sense of fun. Keep yourself on track.

And we have some good news for you: There are changes coming in Phase III and Week 7 that you might like. But don't you dare read ahead until you have finished Week 6.

1. Celebration: You have made incredible progress. Are you feeling more power over food? Are you feeling the food industry's grip on your weakening? Are you starting to notice changes in your body and your measurements? Are you, in fact, starting to feel better about *yourself*?

2. Note from the Doctor: Only 12 percent of all adults in the United States are metabolically healthy, meaning that they don't have diabetes, obesity, elevated lipids (cholesterol and triglycerides), or hypertension. These illnesses are directly linked to the food that we eat and have only become significant in the last 40 years. The severity of COVID-19 is directly related to having any of these

chronic metabolic illnesses. The more of these you have, the higher the risk of respiratory symptoms, an uncontrolled immune response, and death.

Start to notice what has happened to you in just the last five to six weeks. You have improved your sugar, weight, lipids, and blood pressure all while reducing or eliminating medications. You have more energy and alertness. Your skin is starting to glow. Your joints don't hurt as much, or at all. People are noticing that there is a shine in your eyes and that you are looking leaner. They are starting to ask what it is that you are doing and, without knowing it, you have become a leader. You have become a big part of the solution for curing the slow pandemic of diabetes that is killing us all.

3. Tips for Success

    –   Stay on course. You should be focused on eating as much as you want when it comes to low-carb veggies, Alkagizer smoothies, bitter greens, and high-quality proteins and fats like you might find in meat, fish, poultry, and eggs.

    –   Celebrate your wins. Notice your progress and focus on it. Reach out for support. Order what you want in a restaurant, not what they are trying to feed you.

CHAPTER 6

Phase III: From Summer to Winter

Congratulations! You are two-thirds of the way through this program, and you've probably begun to recognize some improvements in your psychology and your physiology—for example, you may have better energy levels.

You probably started this program with a big primary objective, like losing weight or reversing diabetes. This process can feel like climbing a mountain. You climb and you climb, and the summit doesn't seem to be any closer. But it is closer, every day.

Celebrate the progress you have made so far!

In Week 1, we learned about food psychology, the way we talk to ourselves about food and the way the food manufacturing industry talks to and manipulates us. You became more aware of the way food makes you feel and the reasons you choose to eat the foods you eat. You began to create for yourself a real sense of food freedom: the opportunity to eat what you want, when you want, whenever you want it without feeling guilt as well as the freedom *not* to eat what you really don't want to eat without feeling intense regret or feelings of missing out.

In Week 2, we explored how your health is determined far more by making sure you get enough of the good things than by removing foods from your diet. You came to see how most diets, which focus on taking things away, create a sense of lack and loss, which is emotionally challenging. That's why most diets fail. As you added more nutritious foods to your diet, you probably noticed your cravings began to diminish, and you gained a certain amount of freedom over certain types of foods.

In Week 3, we started to gain freedom from the foods that can often control us and take our freedom away and damage our health. We took a holiday from refined sugar, processed foods, and other foods that we call nonfunctional or nonideal. We hope that you found it easier to give these foods up than you have in the past, because you had improved your nutrition and hydration first. Taking a break from some of those foods may even have given you a feeling of relief; well done.

You successfully completed Phase I of your postdiabetic journey and then entered Phase II with Week 4 and headed into Spring. You learned that Spring is an incredibly important season that your body was designed for but may never have fully experienced because it was constantly processing carbohydrates. We learned about the importance of seasonal rotation, how our bodies have evolved to take advantage of seasonal eating patterns, and the value of cyclical eating. You learned that your body will operate best when it gets the opportunity to do all the jobs, in each of the seasons, that it evolved to do.

We moved on to take a break from fresh fruit and continued to eat all the most powerful and important nutritional substances for our bodies: a wide variety of healthy vegetables and good, healthy proteins that moved your body into fat-burning mode. Beginning in Week 4 and continuing through Week 5 and Week 6, you experimented with taking vacations from substances that don't contribute to your health, such as alcohol, dairy, caffeine, and tobacco. You recentered on your "why." Finally, we invited you to surround yourself with like-minded people who will support and sustain you in your journey toward health.

As we promised at the end of the last chapter, we have an enhancement that you're probably going to enjoy: summer is around the corner, and that's where we're going in Week 7.

WEEK 7

Welcome to Week 7! This week Summer is in the air even if it isn't summer where you are right now. You are two-thirds of the way through your journey and moving from a time of low-glycemic abundance to a period when sugar, in certain forms, comes back into season.

We want you to keep doing what you've been doing in Spring and add a couple of things. First, bring into your diet some healthy root vegetables like carrots and beets. You may also, if you wish, add in some low-sugar, high-antioxidant berries like blueberries and raspberries. Spread those out through the week to give your body a sense of Summer. Your body is sensitive to sugar, so take it easy.

Here's why.

The Pleasure Trap

Eric: Deep in the bush of East Africa, I was hunting again with the Hadza bushmen. The heat was pounding down, and the thorns were shredding my shins. Birds called in the distance. I found myself feeling I had stepped into a time machine and gone back to the earliest times of human history. The bushmen were running around, tracking, looking at things, smelling things they found every now and then. Sometimes they dug up the edible root of a plant.

All of a sudden, they became unbelievably excited. They were about 40 feet away from me, and I couldn't tell immediately what they were excited about. I had seen their reaction to fresh animal tracks—that got them excited and usually made them run really fast. This time, they gathered around a big bush, chattering excitedly and reaching into the bush. I didn't understand what was happening.

I walked over and saw they were picking berries. What I learned later, speaking to the chief through my translator, is that these berries are, like most fruits, very seasonal, which is why they were so excited. This experience was very similar to the Paleolithic fruit hunter we told you about earlier in the book.

These people don't have access to sugar or sweet carbohydrates with any kind of regularity. Nature completely controls their supply, so when it's gone, it's gone. There's no temptation to eat something that isn't there, nothing for them to be missing out on. But the minute Mother Nature brings out these red berries, the bushmen are just as excited as a kid standing outside a candy store on Saturday.

Naturally, given all their excitement, I was curious. Were these berries really that yummy? I grabbed one off the tree. It was about the size of a large grape, orange and red, shaped like a small plum. The bushmen were holding the fruit, squeezing the skin and popping the fruit directly into their mouths. I did exactly what they did. As soon as the fruit popped into my mouth, they burst out laughing because of the look on my face.

I had put something in my mouth that was more sour than any sour candy I had ever eaten as a child. It was so sour, I felt my entire face was being sucked into itself. But somehow the experience was also super pleasurable, and within 15 seconds the sourness turned into the most gorgeous sweetness I had ever tasted. Now I could understand their excitement. Before I even thought about it, I was reaching for another fruit—and then another and another.

This fruit is about 70 percent pit. There's only a small layer of flesh, so there's not very much sugar involved. You have to eat a lot of them to get much energy. Perhaps the most interesting fact, though, is that as soon as we began walking away from the bush, every single one of us wanted more. So much so, in fact, that I watched these hunters of animals become hunters of fruit. They stopped scanning the ground for tracks and started scanning the horizon for bushes with fruit on them.

I realized that I was seeing a real-life demonstration of evolved sugar cravings in action. Our ancestors had very little access to fruits like this on a regular basis, yet the vitamins and minerals they contain are nutritionally important. When they were available, it was really important that they got as much as they possibly could. As we ate that fruit, our pancreas created insulin, and soon we had a little bit of surplus insulin, which created a craving for more sugar, and so we went hunting for more fruit.

We did find more fruit trees, and pretty soon we'd eaten so much that we could barely walk. We just ate and ate and ate. I had that pain in the stomach I had as a kid when I ate too much watermelon. We had "overeaten" for sure.

But as I sat there, belly distended, I reflected: this evolutionary process is a good thing. It made sure we took advantage of summer to consume as much fruit as possible, because winter was coming. Winter in Africa, where we evolved, means long times of drought with very limited availability of food and water. We had to fatten up in summer to prepare for it.

How perfect. We eat some fruit. It causes us to crave more. We eat far more than we need today so that we can prepare for the coming winter.

This evolutionary trait works very well when there is rare, seasonal availability of naturally existing fruit. Yet this otherwise perfect design is at the root of the huge health, diabetes, heart disease, and obesity epidemics we are seeing in modern life.

What Eric experienced with the bushmen is called "the pleasure trap." The food industry is very aware of this little mechanism. They know they can slip a little bit of sugar into whatever food you're eating, and it's going to activate that pleasure trap. That's why you often feel like some sort of sweet after you've had a meal. Knowing how this mechanism operates can give you power over it. If in the future some sugar slips into one of your meals and suddenly you feel a powerful craving, you will know that it was intentionally stimulated and that knowledge alone can help you resist it.

Remember also that if you choose, this week, to eat some berries and then walk away from the metaphorical bush, those cravings likely will kick in pretty strongly. Now that you are in summer, buy a basket of blueberries or blackberries, eat a reasonable number—one or two handfuls—and when the cravings come, be careful not to go too far.

Remember that, in the world of the Hadza, a handful of berries represents a significant amount of effort. After you eat them, it wouldn't hurt you to take a walk around the block to simulate a little of that effort (and to get you away from the rest of the berries!).

How to Eat Fruit

We mentioned earlier that it's best to eat fruit on an empty stomach. Try to do that now. If you eat fruit when your stomach is full, you are introducing a sugary mass to a warm, moist environment that it should pass through quickly—but cannot. The sugars may begin to ferment, producing gas and heartburn in some people.

This problem was really brought home when Eric's father—an expert on human evolution who was skeptical of Eric's early research on food and health—suffered a heart attack.

Luckily, his heart attack was not fatal or even particularly severe. One day, as he was recovering, he experienced sharp chest pains. He called his nurse, and she asked him to tell her about his day. What had he eaten, she asked? Fish and rice, with an orange for dessert. "There's your problem," she said. "The fish and rice is going to slow down the digestive process. If you take a sugary orange and put it on top of that, you've created optimal conditions for fermentation or putrefaction, potentially producing acid reflux or gas buildup." The prescription? An antacid pill.

This led Eric's father to call his son on the telephone. "This is only going to happen one time," he said, "but I am admitting you were right about this one thing."

That line became a family joke—Eric's research into nutritional anthropology and food psychology progressed, and Eric's father ended up making similar phone calls to him over the next few years.

One of the things you are likely to notice in Week 7, after several weeks in Spring, is that foods you have never regarded as sweet have become much sweeter on your tongue than you remember them to be. This means that certain foods, like broccoli, spinach, and other more "bitter" vegetables have probably started tasting a bit sweet to you.

One thing we have to master, since Mother Nature no longer has the power to seasonally control our access to fruit, is the ability to consciously choose to taper down and stop, something our ancestors never had to do.

As you move into the end of this week, taper down your fruit consumption, as if you are mimicking the passing of fruit *out of season* in nature. At the end of the weekend, you will be ready to enter one of the most exciting seasons yet.

1. Celebration: You have completed your first visit to Spring! Well done. And now you are sampling Summer and reintroducing some healthy carbs into your diet. You have probably noticed some real differences in your relationship with food, the way you feel, and your various health measurements. Well done!

2. Note from the Doctor: It took years of excess sugar for your body to finally lose insulin sensitivity and for your blood to become caramelized and sticky. It is amazing how much of a beating your body takes and yet keeps ticking. Adding in some root vegetables and some berries might affect your glucose levels but very little. Stay off the medications even if your glucose levels tick up a little, but I doubt they will. Using willpower is hardest the first few days; making habits over these last several weeks will save you.

3. Tips for Success

   – Gradually move into early summer by adding in some root vegetables like carrots and beets and, perhaps, some high-antioxidant summer berries like blueberries or raspberries. If you do decide to have some berries, be gentle about the quantity, watch for possible cravings, and then taper your way off them toward the end of the week. (This might require some short-term willpower.)

–   If you decide to sample some berries, take it easy and do some movement to simulate the effort that might have gone into collecting those berries in the first place. Pay close attention to your food dialogue and notice if the Food Devil tries to use this as an opening to bring up some old cravings.

WEEK 8

Welcome to Week 8! We've talked a lot about the seasons so far. Evolution shaped us specifically for each of the seasons. In some we thrive; in some we simply survive. In Summer and Fall, as we increase our carbohydrate intake, our body gets a powerful signal that Winter is coming. What that means is we need to prepare for a massive reduction in the availability of food, in terms of both calories and nutritional constituents like vitamins and minerals. In the same way that chipmunks and squirrels know by the change of seasons to store nuts, your body knows to store carbohydrates in the form of fat.

Until recently, the leading cause of death for almost every generation has been starvation. Humans evolved incredibly good mechanisms to avoid starvation during the most difficult times. When we find fruit and root vegetables available late in summer, our bodies get a strong signal that winter is coming and they should prepare. If individuals were not effective and efficient at converting carbohydrates into fat, they would not have survived. Only those who evolved that skill survived—and so that is a skill you inherited. This is why today's human beings are far more effective at storing fat than we need to be in the modern world (because, after all, what we consider "normal" was anything but normal for the last two million years of evolution).

Our bodies also used winter as an opportunity for rehabilitation and repair. Food digestion is an incredibly energy-intensive function. Very often after we eat, we feel tired—that's because your body is sending huge amounts of blood flow to the digestive system to stimulate the digestive process. In the same way that when we conduct maintenance on a factory we shut down the production lines, when it's time to do maintenance on our bodies, we should do the same thing.

We do that by fasting.

When people fast, their bodies go into repair mode. They start burning fat as a primary fuel source, because there are no digested sugars coming into the system. There's a significant amount of research on what happens during a fast, because political prisoners have gone on extended fasts under medical supervision in prisons and hospitals around the world. That research shows us what happens when we fast and how to fast intelligently.

The Strength in Fasting

You may recall that among the first things we asked you to do to begin the transformation you are now on was to increase your intake of water and oxygen. We require air within a few minutes and water within a few days. The question is, how often do we require food? Do we need it every few hours? Do we need it every day? We feel as though we do because food was always an incredibly rare commodity for our ancestors. They lived with a low number of available calories per acre because they were hunter-gatherers for the majority of human existence. As a consequence, when food was available, they tended to want to eat it immediately. There were no instincts around avoiding food—which is what dieting is.

Imagine what it was like when the seasons began to change. Water supplies dried up, plants were dying, and your food supply became scarce. The very first day when your ancestors were unable to effectively hunt or gather must have been uncomfortable, unpleasant, and even a bit frightening.

The big question is: Were they weaker or stronger the next day? Because if they had grown weaker every single day they went without food, that would have led to a low likelihood of survival. So while it may have been unpleasant to be without food for that first day, oddly, they may have found themselves feeling stronger. On the second day they felt even stronger still, because they were forcing their bodies into fat-burning mode—burning stored energy, rather than the carbohydrates they no longer were gathering.

The truth is we don't need food every day to run our basic metabolism and move around. We can go for hours, days, even weeks without food.

> *Eric: I tested Winter on my sixth expedition up Mount Kilimanjaro, a 19,341-foot Tanzanian peak that generally takes four or five days to climb. Three days before we were to summit, I decided that I would fast for the remainder of the climb.*
>
> *I went into Winter by consuming only water and broth. Our guides, not surprisingly, thought I was absolutely insane. However, they knew me quite well from our previous trips together, so they accepted that this was my decision and allowed me to proceed. (Had I been a normal tourist, they would have either refused to lead me up the mountain or insisted that I eat.)*
>
> *The total climb from the starting point is over 16,000 feet, and for many people, the final push to the summit is the hardest day of their lives. You begin the summit climb at 11 P.M. The temperature is minus 4 or 5 degrees Fahrenheit (15 or 20 degrees Centigrade), and the wind is blowing at 43.5 to 62 miles (70 to 100 kilometers) per hour. You are surrounded by darkness, slowly ascending a very steep trail that seems endless, laboring to breathe in an atmosphere with half the oxygen you're accustomed to. Most people lack the energy even to carry their own small camera, asking the guides to do so for them.*
>
> *I have now climbed Mount Kilimanjaro seven times. This trip, the sixth, was by far the easiest. I carried my own weighty*

SLR camera with a 500-millimeter lens. I had not had food for three days, and I felt great. Once again, I was experiencing the truth that I knew: when we give our body a break from the constant carbohydrate diet we feed it, we create a surplus of energy and an environment of healing, an opportunity of restoration and repair.

When fasting, we discover something powerful about our energy. We discover the feeling or illusion that the food we eat today provides the energy we use today. Our bodies are finely tuned energy management and storage machines; we are very capable of storing days, weeks, or even months of energy. Fasting both allows us to see this and allows our bodies to perform yet another set of important evolved functions that are generally prevented by modern living.

Winter Is a Time for Repair

One of the extraordinary adaptations of our body is that it can shift between energy sources—carbohydrates, fats, and proteins—and do so in a discriminating way. When you first begin to fast, the body will burn a mix of roughly 50 percent protein and 50 percent fat. As it begins to consume protein, it does not consume healthy protein. Instead, through a process called "autophagy," or "self-eating," it consumes broken and damaged proteins that may be diseased or could lead to disease. This is a fasting phenomenon. It is the maintenance of bodily nutrition by the breakdown of body tissues.

Lions and cheetahs focus their hunting efforts on the weakest members of the herd which, in turn and following the survival-of-the-fittest concept, keeps the herd healthy and strong. Your body does the same thing. During autophagy, your body "eats" the proteins most likely to contribute to illness and disease and makes way for new, younger, and healthier proteins.

We eat to provide fuel, principally in the form of glucose. Anything that we eat can be converted to glucose, be it carbohydrate

(100 percent conversion), protein (up to 50 percent conversion), or fat (10 percent conversion). Glucose is used immediately by our cells if it can get in (thanks to insulin), and the excess is stored as glycogen in our liver and muscles and/or converted to fat.

In a fasting state, the body has no access to dietary carbohydrate, protein, or fat to convert to sugar, so it has to eat itself using its stored fuel and bodily tissues. There have been a variety of studies on the effects of fasting on the body and, according to Valter Longo, Ph.D., author of *The Longevity Diet*, here is an overview:

> **Day 1:** Your body burns the most available fuel, blood sugar and glucose, in the form of glycogen, which is stored in the liver and muscles.

> **Days 2 and 3:** The body has to convert its protein and fat tissues to glucose, usually in a 50/50 mix. This is important both for the consumption of stored fats and for the process of eliminating older or diseased fat or protein cells. As the need for energy becomes more urgent (no dietary sugars being consumed), the body turns its focus on burning stored fat and proteins in a process known as *autophagy*. The beauty of autophagy is that where healthy cells are able to "protect" themselves from being consumed, older or diseased cells cannot, and they are selected for consumption first. In other words, your body burns the oldest and sickest cells first. This, hand in hand with motivated stem cell production, is about as close as we get to an internal fountain of youth.

> **Day 4 and beyond:** The body switches its focus back to fat (autophagy) and slows down consumption of protein cells and stem cell production is kicked into even higher gear.

Through fast-induced autophagy, the body heals itself, gets rid of damaged cells and tissue, makes new cells and tissue, and at the same time generates enormous amounts of life-sustaining energy. It's really a beautiful thing.

Eric: I was informed one day that I was going to have all my wisdom teeth removed. I wasn't particularly happy with that. I'm not a big fan of invasive surgery. Clearly, if one needs stitches, you should get them, but I prefer not to make holes unnecessarily. If I was going to have my wisdom teeth out, I wanted to know why.

Asking around, I found that in my circle of 30 or so friends, about a third of us are missing teeth in the front of our faces. This may have something to do with our being Canadian and playing ice hockey, but it made me think about what life must have been like for our ancestors. It would have been entirely normal to lose teeth in the trauma of fighting and hunting and just going about life the way they did. Wisdom teeth, then, are designed to grow in and help close up the spaces where we lost teeth. As they come in, they push other teeth forward. But if you put in a denture, or if you do not have dental trauma because you were not a hockey player or a Paleolithic hunter-gatherer, you may run out of space in your jaw and need to have your wisdom teeth removed.

I decided I would indeed have mine out and told my dental surgeon I was ready to book a date. He insisted we needed two dates, because he couldn't take four out at once. The pain and the recovery from two was as much as anyone could handle.

I didn't have that much spare time so I countered, "I don't think you've seen my speaking schedule," I said. "I don't have time for two operations; let's get it all done in one session."

He allowed this but only after making me sign a disclaimer.

After the procedure was over, the surgeon handed me two prescriptions: one for antibiotics and one for painkillers.

"No, thank you," I said.

"No, you need to have these," he insisted.

"Could you explain why?"

"Well, you're going to need these painkillers right now because you're still under local anesthetic. When that wears

off, the pain is going to be so intense that you won't be able to think."

"I'm not really into painkillers," I said.

"Humor me. Take the prescription, fill it, and have the pills on hand in case you need them."

"I'll compromise," I said. "I'll take the prescription and keep it in my wallet. And then I'll bring this piece of paper back to you next week, because I won't fill it. Now tell me about the antibiotics."

"You just had surgery," he said, "so you should take antibiotics."

"Did you wash your hands?" I asked him.

"Yes!"

"Did you wash the tools you used?"

"Yes!"

"Were we in a sterile environment?"

"Yes!"

"Do you suspect there is any reason that I should get an infection?"

"No."

"So what you're asking me to do is take antibiotics as a prophylactic against an infection. I won't do that."

"Okay, but listen," he said. "You still could get an infection."

"I'll make this deal with you. I'll take that second prescription too. I'll keep an eye on the surgery site. If it becomes red and inflamed, I'll fill the prescription and take the antibiotics."

He agreed, and I added, "I'll see you in a week and bring both prescriptions back."

I left his office and went straight back to work at my film studio. The pain was entirely manageable. I talked a little funny in meetings because I had cotton in my mouth, but it was fine. Over the next few days everything felt better.

A week later I went for my scheduled post-op visit. The surgeon looked in my mouth and got a puzzled look on his face.

"When were you here?" he asked me.

"A week ago."

"No, no, no. That's not right." He looks at my chart, and it confirms that I had the surgery a week earlier. "That can't be right."

"Why not?"

"I've been doing this for ten years, and I know precisely what the healing pattern is when we take out these teeth. You were here three weeks ago, based on the healing in your mouth."

"Well," I said, "I was here a week ago, just like it says on the chart."

He walked out to consult his receptionist. When he returned, he looked at me and asked me how I had healed so quickly. That started a fascinating conversation about food, nutrition, medicine and, of course, fasting.

What Eric had done was enter a version of Winter. His fast that had put him in optimal healing mode allowed his mouth to heal, by the doctor's own confirmation, three times faster than it would have otherwise. After he explained what he had done in detail, the surgeon said he would share that information with his other patients.

How does this work?

After three days of fasting, your body begins to produce stem cells. Stem cells are kind of omnipotent: They can turn into any kind of cell—brain cell, heart cell, any kind at all. These cells are the engines of repair within the body, replacing damaged cells the body has cleaned out.

We are big fans of using well-planned, structured fasting to stimulate all this repair and to reset insulin sensitivity. It is not, however, a miracle cure. And a point that many fasting advocates miss is that most people in the Western world may be overfed calories but they are underfed nutrients. If they enter a fast in that condition, they are basically starving themselves. To conduct a fast effectively, you have to top up all your nutritional needs so that your body is prepared for a fast in the same way our ancestors prepared for winter.

Winter Is Here

Winter is here, but it comes with options.

Our challenge for you, in Week 8, is to sample winter by attempting a short (three-day) fast. We have offered two formats for you to choose from. We will get to those shortly.

Alternatively, if you don't want to sample Winter, then it is time for you to move straight back to Spring, which means taking another break from carbs and focusing your efforts on green veggies, high-quality proteins, intentional movement, water, and breathing exercises.

If you are ready to try Winter, you have two choices.

The first is hardcore Winter: a water-only fast.

The second is a softer version of Winter in which you consume raw green vegetables, such as the Alkagizer Smoothie, and water.

Your first decision is whether you want to pursue the hardcore or softer version of Winter. Then you need to decide a timeframe: How long will you fast? It's important to make this decision before you begin. If you make the decision on a day-to-day basis, you will torture yourself every day, wondering, *Should I stop today? Should I eat today or not?* Instead, decide on the minimum number of days you will fast. We recommend three days, but we would be proud if you tried one day or two days. We would be thrilled to see you throw yourself into the program at any level.

If you would like to go longer than three days, we recommend going to a health center that specializes in fasting so that you can have the support, massage, and environment that will make it easier.

For now, we recommend going in Winter for at least one full day and up to three full days. Even if you've made it to your minimum number of days, you can always add more days if you are feeling fantastic and want to continue. In the same vein, do not subtract days if you find fasting difficult. Don't quit. The harsh truth is that day one is often unpleasant, and day two can be even more so. Most people feel fantastic by day three.

Now, if you choose to go into Winter, we highly recommend that you discuss this with your doctor and consider getting your measurements updated. (If your doctor tries to dissuade you from fasting, please seek a second medical opinion.)

Once you've chosen a format—just water or water plus greens (and you can add greens later if you like)—and the length of the fast, stick with the following key principles.

Key Principles of Fasting

1. Start your fast in the morning. In other words, simply don't have breakfast. Wake up and have water or water and greens.

2. Stay hydrated. Make sure you are constantly putting water in your system.

3. Be gentle on yourself. Don't travel excessively and avoid driving or operating heavy machinery.

4. Pamper yourself. This is an outstanding week to undertake some gentle yoga classes, go for light walks, get a massage, and go for a steam or sauna.

5. Avoid situations where you will smell food. Strong-smelling foods will stimulate digestive fluid production in your stomach, and that will feel unpleasant.

6. The fast finishes on the morning of the first day after the fast. So if you start your fast on Monday and want to fast for three days, you will break the fast on Thursday morning.

When the time comes to break your fast, do so gently. You will face the classic situation in which your eyes are bigger than your stomach. Because you will not have eaten for anywhere from one to three days, your stomach will have shrunk back to its normal size. Your pancreas will have reset to a glucagon-producing role. You have put your body in a position to respond correctly to small doses of food. So give it small doses of Spring foods.

We will be going from Winter to Spring, so begin with a light meal, such as a small salad or a vegetable stir-fry. Moving into your second meal, add in some healthy fatty proteins like wild-caught salmon. Ease your way back into Spring with gentle eating. Don't end your fast with gluttony. Your body may think it wants that because it thinks you're starving, but you know you are not.

1. Celebration: You are learning and experiencing so much now. You have completed two-thirds of the program and are making some serious progress.

2. Note from the Doctor: Studies are beginning to show the power of fasting in a medical setting. Some cancer patients who fasted for three to five days prior to chemotherapy treatments showed markedly better outcomes. They could tolerate higher doses of chemotherapy with far less intensive side effects. Cancer cells are young and dumb and lack protective skills compared to normal cells, which have an amazing, innate ability to protect themselves in a fasted state. That makes the cancer cells more vulnerable to chemotherapy and the normal cells less vulnerable.

    There's also research showing that diabetics who go on prolonged medically supervised fasts several times a year have been able to reset their sensitivity to insulin and become postdiabetic! Fasting speeds the process of resetting insulin sensitivity. We find all this research very exciting.

3. Tips for Success: This week you have two main choices: Winter or Spring.

    – Hardcore Winter: A water-only fast for between one and three days that then transitions back into Spring.

    – Softer Winter: A water-and-greens fast for between one and three days that then transitions back to Spring.

- Spring: Return to Spring and see how your body feels in Spring for the second time.

- Pick your path. If you choose Winter, choose how many days in advance and be willing to add days but not to subtract any. Also, break the fast in the morning; every night of sleep during the fast is valuable to the healing process.

WEEK 9

Welcome to Week 9! This is the last week of the official program, but it's the first week of the rest of your life during which you will have higher levels of food freedom and a significantly improved health trajectory. This week you're going to be back in Spring, but we're going to show you that there are two versions of Spring.

We are aware that this might not excite you. But we are hoping that your *progress* does excite you.

For some people, Spring feels boring. There can be a lack of variety, and until you learn the different ways to cook and shop, Spring can be challenging. Give yourself credit in this moment, though. Look back at how much change and improvement you have made in your physiology and your food psychology in just eight weeks. Look back at how much progress you've made in undoing the teaching you received over your lifetime from the food industry.

Think about how long your previous lifestyle contributed to where you were when you started this book. If you had been eating for, say, 10 years on a standard modern diet, that's more than 500 weeks during which you taught your body to store carbohydrates as fat and to overproduce insulin. If you've been eating this way for 20 years, that's over 1,000 weeks. Thirty years? Fifteen hundred weeks of training. You've only been doing this program for eight weeks, yet you've already been able to achieve meaningful reversal and repair of the damage done over the last 500 or more weeks. Well done. Keep up the great work.

Also worth considering is the concept of health trajectory. What kind of life are you headed for now compared to three months ago? Every time you make a food decision, you are choosing a "heath direction," and over the last eight weeks, you have taken major steps in the right direction.

The Two Springs

As we head into Week 9, you are going to choose between two kinds of spring:

1. Deep Spring
2. Normal Spring

You should choose which Spring experience you want to continue with based upon your present circumstances and goals.

For instance, if you still have a significant amount of weight to release, or if your blood sugar numbers are far from ideal, you might want to choose to do this week in Deep Spring, just as you have done before.

On the other hand, if you feel like weight loss is not an issue and your blood sugar numbers are in or entering the postdiabetic range, you might want to choose Normal Spring.

Where Normal Spring is different from Deep Spring is that it is probably closer to the truly natural spring season where there would have been access to some occasional carbs. So where you would continue to focus on the same foods and activities as in Deep Spring (veggies; greens; high-quality proteins like eggs, fish, meat and poultry; and some nuts and seeds), you might also add some of the carb-rich veggies like carrots, beets, and other root vegetables like sweet potatoes. You would not, however, want to eat things like pasta, bread, or sugar.

The second thing you're going to look at is your blood sugar numbers. One of our goals here is to get your insulin sensitivity back on track. If you find that you are able to eat a certain quantity of root vegetables and your blood sugar levels do not rise, you may find in another week that you can eat even more of those same root vegetables and your blood sugar levels still do not rise. They may even fall. This is because you are redeveloping and healing your insulin sensitivity. In other words, you are becoming more effective at processing sugar.

On the other hand, if you find that your blood sugar numbers are going up, that indicates you still lack insulin sensitivity. Your system is not yet working properly. If that happens, you might want to go back into Deep Spring, or at least reduce the quantity of root vegetables you eat until your blood sugars come down in a corresponding way.

This low carb intake keeps you in Spring, or ketosis, and allows you to continue your journey, whether that's losing weight, improving your blood sugar numbers, or both.

Your first step is deciding which version of Spring you want to follow. But then you may wonder: *Am I trapped in Spring for the rest of my life? Will I never be able to simply enjoy food again?*

You are not trapped in Spring for the rest of your life!

This entire program is about repairing your body so it can process sugars correctly. You're in Spring right now because doing so helps your body heal and recover. In the following chapter, we provide specific guidelines and strategies for how you can infuse these principles into your life and maintain your good health once you recover it. For now, know that Spring is the healthiest place you can be as you turn your condition around. We know it can feel a bit boring or limiting, but it will pay off and help you return to a life where your body is working well and your relationship with food is back on track.

Have You Made Progress?

Here in Week 9, you're probably in one of two camps. In the first camp, you've had a phenomenal recovery. You may already be postdiabetic. You may have lost weight, changed your relationship with food, and now know with certainty that your destiny is altered and your health has been dramatically improved.

Or you're in the second camp. You're not certain you are getting results. You're thinking, "Wow, I'm eight weeks in, I've been paying attention, and I just don't feel like I'm experiencing the level of recovery I need to experience." If that is the case, remember how long it took to create the health conditions in the first place. Remember, too, that progress is incredibly hard to witness when you are close to it—parents have trouble seeing their children's incremental growth, for example, until they take them clothes shopping. When change is happening incrementally in front of you day by day, it's hard to see. But if you come back a week or two later, you'll notice it. Come back a year later, and the results are dramatic. If you're in this camp and you feel like progress isn't as dramatic as you'd like, we get it!

Now is the time to take a good look at the indicators and measurements you've been tracking for the last eight weeks—blood sugar levels, blood pressure, weight, physical measurements. You are likely to see slight, incremental improvements. Don't just look at last week. Go back to the beginning of the program. How has your weight been affected? How has your body fat percentage been affected? How has your physical size been affected compared to now?

If you've come this far and you believe what we have taught you has not worked, then we are desperate to hear from you. Please go to **http://www.postdiabetes.com/links/readersurvey** and fill out this anonymous survey. We want to find out what worked well and what could be better and how we can support you in getting the results you want.

On the other hand, if you feel our program does work for you—well, we want to hear from you too. At **http://www.postdiabetes .com/links/readerstories**, you can share your successes and show us your results.

Your answers to both of these surveys will help us improve what we teach. What you share will be an enormous help not only to us but also to tens of thousands of other people like you who need and want to get better.

You're well equipped now to head into your new, healthier life. Before you do, though, we are going to share some additional insights about how to think about food.

1.   Celebration: At this point, your healing journey is well underway. You might have already transitioned beyond diabetic concerns. Perhaps you've shed some pounds, transformed your bond with nutrition, and now firmly believe that your future is reshaped and your well-being has significantly enhanced. Applaud yourself for committing to this regimen and placing your health at the forefront.

2.   Tips for Success: This week you have two main choices now: Deep Spring or Normal Spring.

     –   Deep Spring: veggies; greens; high-quality proteins like eggs, fish, meat and poultry; and some nuts and seeds.

     –   Normal Spring: veggies; greens; high-quality proteins like eggs, fish, meat and poultry; and some nuts and seeds. You might also add some of the carb-rich veggies like carrots, beets, and other root vegetables like sweet potatoes. You would not, however, want to eat things like pasta, bread, or sugar.

3.   Now is the time to take a good look at the indicators and measurements you've been tracking for the last eight weeks—blood sugar levels, blood pressure, weight, and physical measurements. You are likely to see slight, incremental improvements. Don't just look at last week. Go back to the beginning of the program. How has your weight been affected? How has your body fat percentage been affected? How has your physical size been affected compared to now?

PART III

SUSTAINING YOUR POSTDIABETIC JOURNEY

Rubén: If you're reading this section, it means one of two things. You're either the kind of person who turns to the last part before you buy a book, or you've read everything that came before. Maybe you even adhered to our admonition and didn't read ahead as you progressed week by week through the program. You may even be postdiabetic by now. And you may be asking yourself: Where do I go from here? What do I eat? How do I stay on track? How can I get my kids and my friends and co-workers to live a healthier life as well, if only because it will make things easier for me?

This chapter answers those questions. In the next few pages, Eric provides guidelines from his work with WILDFIT to help you live the most optimal, healthy version of yourself indefinitely into the future.

+ + +

Eric: I am really excited for you. When you picked up this book, you may have felt trepidation or concern, but you also believed that you could reverse type 2 diabetes if you were willing to buy it, read it, and follow it. You may feel, now that you are on the other side of your nine-week journey, that you are at the end.

You're not.

In fact, you are beginning an entirely different destiny—one in which you get to have a different relationship with food and the food manufacturing industry. As a result of that, you also get to have a different relationship with the medical industry. What we hope is that, because of the turnaround that you have created in yourself, you are able to live a long, prosperous, healthy, wonderful life. In order for you to do that, I am going to share with you the core principles and strategies that make WILDFIT's coaching programs so effective.

My experience in 1991 of healing my ill health through diet was the genesis of everything that would become WILDFIT. Over the next ten years, I undertook deep research into two core areas: evolutionary nutrition and behavioral change psychology. I wanted to know what people should really be eating, and why they don't, even when they know they should.

WILDFIT has become incredibly successful. At the time of this writing, we have served over 50,000 people in 130 countries. Largely, these people found us by word of mouth because they saw the results that their friends were getting and decided to try WILDFIT for themselves. To introduce you to what we do, here are the core teachings that make WILDFIT effective, not only as a health transformation program but also as a lifestyle.

Congratulations on successfully laying the groundwork for a healthier, postdiabetic future! As you embark on the next phase of your journey, it's essential to have the right tools and resources to maintain your newfound wellness. In this part of the book, we will equip you with the knowledge and guidance you need to stay on track and continue reaping the benefits of your lifestyle transformation.

In the chapters that follow, we will delve into the fundamentals of a well-balanced, nutritious diet that will support your ongoing health goals. We'll start by discussing the foods that should form the cornerstone of your meals and explore the Four Food Classes that can help you create a diversified and enjoyable eating plan. We'll then guide you through the process of combining these classes and adapting your diet according to the seasons, ensuring that you make the most of the natural variety available throughout the year.

Next, we'll introduce you to the WILDFIT ratios, a strategic approach to the WILDFIT seasons that can optimize your energy levels and overall well-being. We'll also discuss the WILDFIT principles, which serve as a compass for making informed decisions about your food choices, ultimately supporting your long-term health.

Finally, we'll provide you with actionable tips and strategies to help you stay on track with your new lifestyle. From setting realistic goals and tracking your progress to navigating social situations and cultivating a supportive network, we'll ensure that you're well prepared to face the challenges and embrace the rewards of your postdiabetic journey.

As you read through these chapters, remember that lasting change takes time, patience, and perseverance. Equip yourself with the knowledge and tools provided in this part of the book, and you'll be well on your way to a sustainable, healthy future— one that is free from the constraints of diabetes.

CHAPTER 7

What Should I Eat Now?

We can start to answer that question by asking, "What is food?" The dictionary definition is "any nutritious substance that people or animals eat or drink in order to maintain life and grow; nourishment, provisions."[1]

What makes a particular food nutritious? There are things that are nutritious for one species but not for another. Then there are things that are nutritious to one species and, in fact, lethal to another. The tamboti tree in sub-Saharan Africa is regular fare for the black rhino but would cause illness or death for us.

There are also different classifications for "nutritious"—we require both energy and non-energy nutrients in our diet. In fact, it might be useful to consider the various kinds of nutrients that your body requires and/or utilizes.

AMINO ACIDS

Many people focus on getting enough protein; we recommend being aware that what you really require is a combination of 20 amino acids in order to build the various proteins our bodies require. Proteins are large and often complex molecules that perform a variety of jobs in the body; examples include insulin and antibodies.

A healthy human can manufacture 11 of the required amino acids but the other 9* are considered essential and must be obtained through the consumption of food that contain them.

While amino acids can be obtained from both plant- and animal-based foods, the proteins found in animal products are more complete and contain all the essential amino acids we require.

FATTY ACIDS

We get fatty acids by consuming fat, the best sources being from animal fats. Yes, we need fat. As we have discussed, fat has been unfairly demonized by the sugar industry, and while there are clearly poor-quality fats (trans fats) to avoid, most of us would benefit from increasing our intake of healthy, naturally occurring fats.

Fat is quite rare in nature; our ancestors prized it, and we evolved powerful cravings for it.

CARBOHYDRATES

We eat and burn carbohydrates as quick-burn energy. If we eat more than we can burn, we store the excess energy as glycogen (in the liver or muscles) or as fat. There is of course a spectrum of available carbohydrates, ranging from "healthy on occasion" to disastrous, with fresh fruit at one end of the scale and refined sugar and flour at the other.

Carbohydrates, like fat, are also quite rare in nature, but rather than being constantly rare, they range from seasonal abundance to complete absence, depending upon the season. As we have discussed, our bodies have adapted to handle these extremes but not the extreme and constant access to carbohydrate foods we face today.

---

*   The nine essential amino acids are histidine, isoleucine, leucine, lysine, methionine, phenylalanine, threonine, tryptophan, and valine (https://www.healthline.com/nutrition/essential-amino-acids).

VITAMINS

Vitamins are organic molecules that our bodies need to perform a variety of functions and to maintain general health. There are 13 currently known required vitamins[†] that we cannot synthesize on our own and must, therefore, get them from our food. They are therefore considered essential.

MINERALS

Minerals are inorganic substances (or chemical elements) that occur naturally in soil and water. They are absorbed by plants and then absorbed by herbivores (who eat the plants) and again by omnivore and carnivore species. They are, of course, returned to the soil and water as waste products or when the organism at the top of the food chain dies and decomposes.

There are at least 20 chemical elements[2] required by the body to support biochemical processes, provide structure, or use as electrolytes. Some of these elements are required in large quantities, and others are required in trace quantities only.

We require food for both building blocks (vitamins, minerals, amino acids) and energy sources (fats, carbohydrates). Our bodies have evolved both these nutritional requirements and the ability to extract these nutrients from certain foods.

Wood, for instance, probably does contain nutrients required by people, but as we have not evolved either the teeth or digestive processes to break it down, wood is not a good source of nutrients as far as humans are concerned.

For most of our history, our diet was influenced by two major factors: what nature provided and our evolved cravings. Today, we can pretty much eat anything we want (in any quantity), and our own cravings are being used against us to boost profits for food manufacturers.

These days, our food contains very little naturally occurring essential nutrients and too much surplus energy. One result of this

---

[†]   The 13 essential vitamins are vitamins A, C, D, E, K, and the B vitamins: thiamine (B_1), riboflavin (B_2), niacin (B_3), pantothenic acid (B_5), pyroxidine (B_6), biotin (B_7), folate (B_9) and cobalamin (B_{12}).

is that most people are eating too much energy and not enough essential nutrients. They are both overfed and malnourished at the same time.

As a reminder, our bodies were designed to take advantage of seasonal abundance of carbohydrate foods for a few weeks or months at a time. Our bodies take the abundance of carbs as a cue that drought is on the way. The more we eat, the more glycogen and fat we store. It is not difficult to imagine what would happen to someone who ate like this for years at a time.

Further, the quality of carbs we are being assaulted with has to be taken into account. The Western tendency is to eat foods that are incredibly rich in calories and contain additives like corn syrup and other types of sugar that lead to reduced insulin sensitivity and increased risk of type 2 diabetes. This is a major factor in both the diabetes and obesity epidemics.

Let's also talk about one of the most ridiculous ideas to come out of the field of nutrition: *the recommended daily allowance.*

Our species evolved to survive seasonal fluctuations and food availability. Accordingly, our bodies have learned to store many nutrients so there is no need to consume them every day or even every week. For example, vitamins A, D, E, and K are stored in your fatty tissues, and vitamin B_{12} is stored in your liver, so you don't need to ingest these five vitamins as often as you need to consume the water-soluble vitamins like vitamin C.

Another important consideration related to seasonal fluctuation is that our bodies also get messages from our food. As we have discussed, carbohydrate foods suggest to the body that winter is coming and that the body should burn less dietary sugar and store more of it. The result? Insulin sensitivity problems and weight gain.

We should also consider the "non-nutrition" foods that our bodies need.

WATER

While some will argue that water is not a nutrient per se, it really is an essential nutrient in that we can't survive more than a few days without it. While water does, often, contain nutrients (minerals), it is also a building block that our bodies use to manufacture tissue.

FIBER

While we don't derive much nutritional satisfaction directly from fiber, it has been shown to support the growth of gut bacteria.

If a food does not meet at least one of these requirements, it isn't really a food. If it meets some of the requirements but we have not evolved the ability to digest and extract value from it, it's still not a food to us. (As we discussed, wood is nutritious to beavers and termites, but not to humans.) This point is important; we are constantly being told that various "foods" have been fortified in some way, but none of that speaks to whether our bodies are able to extract and process that fortification. We advocate getting your nutritional needs met from the best and most complete natural food sources first.

We evolved certain nutritional dependencies and food processing capacities. Our proper human diet is made up of foods that lie at the intersection of dependencies and capacities.

We use this logic to classify modern foods into four classes. Remember food freedom? These classes are essential to achieving it.

CHAPTER 8

The Four
Food Classes

We borrow these food classifications from Eric's company, WILD-
FIT. The idea is not to create a dictatorial food classification system
but rather a guideline of organizing principles that you can use to
classify food *for yourself*.

For instance, if you are, today, dealing with type 2 diabetes,
we might suggest that you avoid entirely white rice and place it in
class 4. Later, once you are postdiabetic, you might move it up to
class 3 and enjoy it from time to time.

To start, there are two classifications of *functional* foods and
two classifications of nonfunctional food. Class 1 foods are considered essential; we have a longstanding relationship with them
and certain nutritional dependencies on them. Class 2 foods are
also functional but not essential; they may be "healthy," but they
are not specifically necessary. Classes 3 and 4 are nonfunctional
and are foods that should be avoided or consumed occasionally.

Here they are in more detail.

CLASS 1: ESSENTIAL FOODS

Healthy green vegetables; seasonally available fruit; lean, high-
quality proteins such as ethically raised meats, fish, shellfish, and

eggs; and nuts and seeds. Some of these foods (meats, fishes, eggs) can be eaten almost year-round, whereas the plant-based foods should be consumed with more seasonal rotation.

These foods are considered essential and must be consumed in appropriate quantities.

CLASS 2: OPTIONAL FOODS

These aren't really necessary, but there are no downsides to them so long as you don't overindulge. These are foods you could never argue are required to maintain health—for example, avocados. They are from South America; we have no evolved relationship with them, as our ancestors had no access to them. But they're full of folic acid and healthy fats, so even though they're not legacy human foods, they can be quite beneficial.

Stop here.

The only real "food" for humans are Class 1 and Class 2 foods; everything else is really a nonfood. That is to say that it is edible, but the benefit of eating it does not outweigh the potential harm.

Eating nonfoods creates several challenges.

- First, nonfoods and junk foods displace healthy foods, as you have less appetite for them.

- Second, nonfoods are often very high in low-quality calories, which cause both short- and long-term blood sugar issues and may lead to the development of type 2 diabetes, obesity, and food addiction.

- Third, nonfoods often lack water content, which means the body has to use its own water to digest them, leading to dehydration.

- Fourth, nonfoods often contain substances our bodies are not capable of processing effectively, which leads the body to use additional energy to process them and to reject unwanted substances. Nonfoods can cause increased toxicity, allergic reactions, and stress the immune system.

CLASS 3: NONFUNCTIONAL OCCASIONAL CONSUMPTION

These are foods that you might enjoy for emotional reasons. Since you know that they are not ideal, it is a good idea to only consume them from time to time.

Remember that you might have a food that you *know* should be Class 4 (nonfood), but you are just not ready to totally give it up yet. No problem: most Class 3 foods are, in a sense, auditioning for Class 4.

CLASS 4: NONFOODS

What we consider to be Class 4 foods and what you consider to be Class 4 foods may be different. But they have one thing in common: you never eat them; you just don't see them as food.

It's up to you to determine what these foods are, but here's how you know: when you are offered this food, your response is not, "Oh, I wish I could," or "Not today." Your response is, "No, thanks; I don't eat that." You just don't see it as an option, and, of course, it doesn't require any willpower to avoid.

Your definition of Class 4 foods will mature and refine over the years. Right now there may be foods you are not ready to say good-bye to. You might want to have them occasionally. But you may come to realize how good you feel when you don't eat them, because the healthier you get, the more honest your body becomes with you and you with it, the more foods you will move into Class 4.

How you classify foods is up to you. You're going to do that when you want to, not because we came along and told you to. But when you do these things—when you recognize and live by these food categories for yourself—that's when you empower yourself with food freedom to eat what you want, as much as you want, when you want, whenever you want to eat it.

CHAPTER 9

Combining Classes & Seasons

You might be thinking, "Wait a minute. I understand you don't want to tell me exactly what to eat and what not to eat, but can't you give me a hint? Can't you tell me what's in each category?"

To navigate food classes optimally, first you have to think about food classifications. Then, overlay that concept on your eating seasons: WILDFIT Summer, Fall, Winter, and Spring.

Summer is a season of growth and abundance. (No matter where you are when you are reading this book—whether you're in Yellowknife or Copenhagen or Moscow—remember that the Summer we describe is not your summer: it is the summer of sub-Saharan Africa, where 99 percent of human evolution took place.) There is ample sunlight, significant quantities of water, plant life, and animals for hunting. There is limited availability of root vegetables and occasional berries. If your blood sugar levels are healthy, you should be able to live in and enjoy Summer without spiking them.

The majority of the carbohydrates you eat during Summer are "slow" carbs (principally plant-based foods), meaning that the body needs time and effort to extract the sugars inherent in them. If you have functional insulin sensitivity, you would not see significant blood sugar fluctuations during Summer. If your insulin sensitivity is reduced, you may see some blood sugar spikes until that sensitivity is repaired.

One of the ways our body adapts to Summer is that when it eats carbohydrates, it looks for more because it recognizes that loading up on carbs now may make the difference when it comes time to survive winter. Eating carbohydrates, as you know, creates a craving to eat more.

Fall is the season of caloric abundance and comes very naturally after summer. Summer carbs stir the cravings and then fall abundance kicks in; root veggies, honey, and fruit are suddenly more abundant. There are still plenty of plants and animals available. This season can run from moderate to high-glycemic, depending on how long you let the season last.

As you now know, when we eat carbohydrates, we burn what we need immediately—they're like working capital for the body, cash flowing in and out. If there is excess, the body burns those carbohydrates and stores them in the muscles as glycogen—the equivalent of a short-term deposit at the bank. If your body needs those carbohydrates, the pancreas creates glucagon to break down the glycogen and withdraw those deposits. But if you continue to eat and your glycogen stores are full, then the body begins making long-term energy storage deposits in fat tissue, preparing you for Winter.

In **Winter** (represented for our ancestors as long dry periods of drought) our bodies can be forced (by lack of food) to switch fuel sources away from carbs and fat to protein. This is an exciting time and is why smart fasting can be such a good idea.

When your body starts consuming proteins for energy, it is part of a process called autophagy, and it truly is brilliant. Your body does not just randomly burn any proteins it can find; it seeks out the old, sick, and weak proteins and burns them first. This is an important function of the body that most people in the Western world are completely missing out on.

Spring is a magical time for the body. With Winter winding down, the rains start, and a new cycle of abundance begins. New plants shoot up and hunting gets easier. We move into a season that triggers ketosis (fat burning) to help you burn off any fat left over from Winter.

In WILDFIT, we speak of three versions of Spring:

1. **Traditional Spring**, which can be very helpful in losing weight and resetting insulin sensitivity. During Spring, we recommend avoiding almost all carbs and increasing your intake of healthy proteins and fats while continuing to eat a wide variety of low-carb veggies. (In the future, once insulin sensitivity has been repaired, you may be able to enjoy a "lighter" version of Spring, with up to 25 grams of high-quality carbohydrates and stay in ketosis.)

2. **Hunter's Spring**, which is a short period of time on a meat-only or meat-prioritized program. This means focusing on the highest-quality, ethically raised nose-to-tail animal products, including meat, fish, eggs and organ meats. (Check out our video on Hunter's Spring for more information.*)

3. **Gatherer's Spring** is a version of Spring that does not include any animal products. Because there are certain nutrients (amino acids, fats, and vitamins) that are more difficult to attain in the absence of animal products, we suggest reviewing our guide to Gatherer's Spring.†

In summary, the purpose of Summer and Fall is to build up energy stores; Winter is an opportunity for repair and recovery; and Spring is an opportunity to reset insulin sensitivity, release excess fat, and begin the process again.

---

* www.GetWILDFIT.com/aboutspring-hunters

† www.GetWILDFIT.com/aboutspring-gatherers

CHAPTER 10

WILDFIT Ratios

Without nature moving us through the seasons, you have to make your own decisions about how long to stay in each one. We've created the WILDFIT ratios to help you do that. These ratios are the number of days you should plan to spend in each season, depending on your goals.

For example, if you have the goal of preparing for an endurance race, you might do a season of Summer and one of Fall in the weeks leading up to the race in order to build up energy stores. But shortly prior to the race, you might do a brief bout of Winter, followed by Spring. That allows you to build up energy and prepare for a long, slow release of that energy through the race.

On the other hand, you might have the goal of losing weight. In that case, you'd want a large number of days set in Spring and Winter. Someone trying to increase insulin sensitivity would employ a similar strategy.

For example, someone looking to lose weight or repair insulin sensitivity issues might want to use a ratio like this:

Summer-Fall-Winter-Deep Spring

3-2-3-23

Three days of Summer, two days of Fall, three days of Winter (fasting), and then twenty-three days in Deep Spring

On the other hand, someone who has achieved postdiabetic status and has arrived at their ideal body weight/composition might choose this:

Summer-Fall-Winter-Spring

20-5-3-3

Twenty days of summer, five days of Fall, three days of Winter, and three days of Spring

CHAPTER 11

Core WILDFIT Principles

PRINCIPLE 1: SAY NO TO DIETS

The origin of the word *diet* is fascinating. In its earliest usage, *diet* meant "lifestyle." It meant "way of life." It was not a temporary alteration to your eating pattern so you could fit into a particular outfit for a special occasion. This is an incredibly important principle because as long as people think of a diet as a temporary change, they are never going to make a permanent shift in their lifestyle. What we do at WILDFIT is about making substantive changes to your relationship with food and with your body.

PRINCIPLE 2: EVERY LIVING THING ON EARTH HAS A SPECIFIC DIET AND EVOLVED FOOD-PROCESSING ABILITIES AND DEPENDENCIES

If you ever watch a nature program, you hear the narrator say something like, "The elephant eats 440 pounds (200 kilograms) of bark and grass and drinks 70 gallons of water every day." The narrator won't be specific whether this elephant is in Tanzania or

India, because elephants the world over are pretty much the same in this regard.

Understand that evolution is a painfully slow process. A species like *Homo sapiens* needs hundreds of thousands of years to evolve meaningful changes to our digestive system. This gives us a powerful clue as to what our diet is and where it evolved (Africa).

Beyond nutrition, many of the body's organs have dual functions; if we don't allow those functions to be exercised, we run the risk of injury or disease.

PRINCIPLE 3: THE MORE CLOSELY ANY LIVING THING ADHERES TO ITS EVOLVED DIET, THE MORE HEALTH AND LESS DISEASE IT WILL EXPERIENCE

When a plant or animal is living the way it evolved to live, it tends to live longer, be healthier, recover from injury more quickly, and fight off or recover from diseases much more effectively.

When an organism moves off its diet, it runs a number of risks, including becoming malnourished or developing some sort of imbalance or even toxicity buildup or poisoning—all of which are prevalent in our society today.

The reason you're reading this book is that human beings took a significant left turn away from our traditional relationship with sugar, which is why, over the last 30 years, diabetes numbers have exploded. This wasn't simply about eating the wrong things—it was eating too much of the right thing at the wrong times, compared to how we evolved.

PRINCIPLE 4: HEALTHY FOOD DOES NOT FIGHT DISEASE; ITS ABSENCE WILL CAUSE OR CONTRIBUTE TO THE DEVELOPMENT OF DISEASE

We live in a culture where people talk about food being medicine. This is a common misconception. In order for your body to do what it needs and wants to do, it doesn't require medicine. It requires that its nutritional needs be met. As long as we think of food as medicine, we tell ourselves we can do what we want to do until we get sick, then eat the right food and recover. This is wrong. What we need to be doing every single day is seeking out the best possible hydration and broad-spectrum nutrition that we can to maintain our health. The first mission must be to get our nutritional needs met.

PRINCIPLE 5: HUMANS EVOLVED TO SURVIVE SEASONAL ROTATION AND CYCLICAL AVAILABILITY OF FOOD AND WATER

Our species, like all species, evolved to survive. In our case, we adapted to seasons and food cycles so that our nutritional requirements are met over a period of time. Suggestions that there is some perfect combination of vitamins and minerals that every human should eat every day are absurd. The only things that should be listed as daily requirements are oxygen and water. Food, on the other hand, should be eaten in a variety of periods and seasons.

PRINCIPLE 6: THE FOOD MANUFACTURING AND MARKETING INDUSTRY IS NOT ON YOUR SIDE

We can't trust them. Food manufacturers are, like any company, driven by profits. They seek to increase profits by selling more food and lowering their costs. The net result of this is that most people are overfed and undernourished. Food manufacturers create marketing campaigns and include addictive ingredients, both tactics designed to get people to eat far more food than they require. Unlike tobacco companies, they are manipulating a basic requirement of life—food—to generate increased profits, and in so doing causing a massive healthcare crisis. They are not above spending phenomenal sums of money to influence governments through lobbying activities to boost their profits even further.

PRINCIPLE 7: "EVERYTHING IN MODERATION" INCLUDES YOUR HEALTH AND LONGEVITY

When people say, "everything in moderation," they generally are trying to justify eating nonfunctional foods. A moderate diet will result in moderate health, which is why the two largest killers in the world, heart disease and cancer, are generally regarded as "lifestyle diseases" when, really, they are "going off the correct lifestyle" diseases.

PRINCIPLE 8: NOTHING TASTES AS GOOD AS GOOD HEALTH FEELS

People often make food decisions in the moment, without realizing the cumulative damage; the short-term pleasure of a tasty treat can be extremely painful and expensive in the long run. When we begin to focus on the long-term quality of life, it becomes much easier to make smart short-term decisions about food.

PRINCIPLE 9: YES, YOU CAN HAVE "TREAT DAYS," BUT TREAT YOURSELF WELL

The idea of a "treat" comes from the concept "to give someone a treat" or to "treat someone well."

The next time you are planning to treat yourself, ask, "Am I going to treat myself well, or am I going to treat myself badly?" Treating yourself doesn't have to involve sugary or fatty foods. You can treat yourself well in much more constructive ways. This can include a trip to the spa, a bike ride, or seeking out foods that feel like a treat but also treat you well.

Remember the rules that you created as a child that defined what a treat is—you were influenced by misguided adults and a manipulative food industry. This is why chocolate has taken over Easter, even though Jesus never ate any. This is why candy canes have taken over Christmas and ice cream has taken over July Fourth and pie has taken over Thanksgiving.

In the end, our rules about treats were bought and paid for. Now it's time for you to make your own.

PRINCIPLE 10: LEADING IS BETTER THAN PUSHING

We all have our own reasons for wanting to bring our friends, families, and co-workers into a healthy lifestyle. The key is not to push but to attract. The healthier you live, the better example you create for others. When you lead by example, people around you will simply arrive at the point where they want to have what you are having. When you try to push somebody, they naturally resist. Instead, be the change that you hope to see in the people you love and the people around you.

Understanding and embracing these principles can help you create lifelong food freedom by truly understanding your relationship with food and empowering you to make significantly better decisions on a daily basis. Remember, it's not the short-term, one-off exceptions that cause disease and difficulty in the future. It's what we do on a daily or regular basis. These principles will help you to create daily rituals, daily beliefs, and daily decisions that lead you toward an incredibly healthy life.

CHAPTER 12

How to Stay
on Track

With those principles understood, let's discuss some of the mental
tips you can use to stay on track.

FOOD PSYCHOLOGY

In Phase I, we focused on food psychology, your inner dialogue,
how you make decisions about what to eat and when to eat it,
and how food makes you feel. We noticed, for example, how an
emotionally charged food can make us feel good even before we
eat it. As we began to understand that food is largely an emotional
journey, we began to pay attention to what is going on mentally
relative to food.

By paying close attention to your food decisions, you can bring
these internal conversations to the forefront of your consciousness. That gives you real opportunity to make improvements and
maintain them for years to come.

Now, keep the game going. If you want something that is a
nonfunctional food, notice what you are saying to yourself, notice how the Food Devil on your shoulder is trying to manipulate
you. The more clearly you understand the Food Devil's sales strategy, the more freedom you can create for yourself. Have you ever

noticed how your Food Devil can sound like a whining teenager? Does your Food Devil sometimes use deals or shame, or use food as a reward? The better you understand the Devil's manipulations, the more power you have to defend yourself.

Recognize Your Hungers

When you are able to slow down and see which of the Six Human Hungers drives your desire, you can address that hunger and make better decisions. Remember, for example, that a dehydrated body may ask for food instead of water because historically we got much of our water through food. The next time you're feeling snacky, start with a big glass of water and see if that changes things.

Having worked with hundreds of thousands of people over the past several years, we have isolated Six Human Hungers that drive all eating decisions. If you need a refresher, please watch this video by Eric to learn more about the hungers and gain more control over your cravings: **www.PostDiabetes.com/links/video-6hungers**.

Notice How You Feel

Remember that most food decisions are about changing the way you feel. Slow down and pay attention to how you feel just before the desire kicks in. How do you feel after you decide to eat something? How about after the first bite? How about after all the other bites? How do you feel an hour later? The next day?

Our food decisions are based on how we're going to feel in the next five minutes. By shifting your consciousness and paying attention to the entire timeline, you're going to recognize that most foods that might make you feel really good in five minutes have later consequences that significantly outweigh that pleasure.

We call this "observing your Food Timeline," and it can really help you become conscious of your food dialogue.

Here is a video of Eric speaking about the good timeline and how you can use it to give yourself food freedom: **www.PostDiabetes .com/links/video-FoodTimeline**

TREAT YOURSELF WELL

Give yourself a treat day. Being overly fanatical about anything is generally a bad idea. There is a difference between the idea of having a treat day on a regular schedule and the approach we prefer, which is treat ratios. For example, you might commit to a 6:1, 10:1, or 28:1 treat ratio. Once you have a treat day, commit to your fixed number of normal days, at a minimum, before you have another treat day. You don't have to have a treat day on the sixth day, for example—but you can.

Remember that treat days are not about treating yourself badly—they are about treating yourself well, as Eric described in Chapter 11 in the WILDFIT Principles.

These tips will help you stay on track by showing that you are not going to live a restricted life. Rather, this is about a sense of freedom. In order to understand the way freedom works, we need to get clear about what that means. Freedom in our world means the freedom to eat what you want, when you want, whenever you want, as much as you want—*and* also to be able to not eat what you don't want to eat when you don't really want to be eating.

THREE REASONS PEOPLE MATTER TO YOUR SUCCESS

The traditional diet industry has failed people. The average person gains three pounds every time they go on a diet. Our success rate at WILDFIT has been phenomenal, and one of the reasons is because we make the community an essential part of the process. One of the things we've discovered by coaching thousands of individuals in over 130 countries around the world is that community is a key component for creating lasting change for people.

There are three primary reasons why the people you spend time with are going to have a major impact on your ability to make the changes you want and to live the life you want.

The first is peer pressure. Not teenage "smoke this cigarette to be cool" peer pressure, but the subtle, unconscious peer pressure that makes us want to fit in with the people around us. The more we love and respect those people, the more we want to fit in. There will come a moment when we are making a food decision, and the unconscious desire to fit in will affect that choice. The more time we spend around people who have healthy habits and similar values around the recovery of long-term health, the better our chances of making a recovery.

This does not mean you must bid good-bye to everyone in your family who enjoys the occasional Big Mac or plate of pancakes. It does mean that you should build a strong social group of people around you that have health as one of their highest values.

Second is the matter of convenience. Food is an incredibly social thing. When we get together as a culture, we do it around food. The next time a friend says, "Want to go grab a bite?", if you are in a healthy social network, you are more likely to make healthy food decisions.

If you don't have a strong support team, if you feel socially alone, you are like the primate suddenly separated from the group in the jungle. You start to feel scared and decide you had better eat anything that is available because your survival is on the line. By maintaining social connections, by spending time with people you love and respect, you create a sense that you are safe. When you feel safe, you will make the very best food decisions for your present and long-term health.

Conclusion

Congratulations on reaching the end of the beginning of your journey to better health and a postdiabetic life! We told you this would not be easy, and we're sure you now know we were not joking. Change is hard, but your results, even if they have been slow in coming, should have revealed to you that change is worth the effort too.

Let us send you on your way with a few thoughts.

First, remember where you came from, because as you're following the principles of this book, you will get better; and as you get better, you will forget how bad things were. It's likely that you will walk into your doctor's office one day and find that you are postdiabetic. It's also likely that if you continue on this path, you one day will drop the word *diabetic* altogether.

Paradoxically, there's risk in that achievement. The more distant your memories of diabetes become, the more distant your memories of the *consequences* of diabetes become. If you are not vigilant, your Food Devil will convince you to make exceptions "just this once."

Remember what life was like before you started this journey. Stay in touch with that feeling. In the future, when you are in those interesting social situations with convenient foods, or you've had a terrible day at work, that memory will help you avoid giving in to the Food Devil. Stand strong by revisiting your records of achievement. Go ahead and read your former BMI and blood sugar numbers in your journal. Look at your "before" pictures—look at them carefully and honestly. Remember who you were. And always reconnect with your "why."

Second, we never want you to feel bad about the food decisions you make. Imagine something momentous happening in your life, and you tell yourself, "What I really need right now is a honey cruller." On a conscious level, you don't need it. Your Food Angel will probably tell you firmly that you don't need it. But if the Food Devil wins this one time, don't feel guilty about it. We want you to feel empowered by letting that event be a lesson to you.

If you eat a Class 4 food that you said you would never, ever eat again, the last thing we want you to do is feel guilty about it, because guilt will create a low emotional state that will drive low-quality eating decisions. Instead, consider what has happened through the principle of failing fast or even of simple experimentation.

In other words, if you've made that decision, make it cleanly. Eat the honey cruller with joy and bliss but stay conscious. Notice how it tastes. Was it as good as you thought it would be? Was the second bite as good as you thought it was going to be? How's that feeling in your mouth afterward? How do you feel half an hour later, or an hour later? Did you sleep well? Are you low energy? Does your stomach hurt a little bit?

If any of those things are true, then you created an incredibly positive result out of your experiment. That result may make it possible for you to move that food back into Class 4 and never think about it again. When you make exceptions, don't think of them as exceptions; think of them as experiments.

Third, as much as your relationship with food is 90 percent of the healing journey, remember that there are other things you can and should do to support that journey. One of them is intentional movement. Make sure that you get some basic movement in every day. You may not enjoy going out and doing exercise. Instead, find excuses, reasons, and motivations to physically move your body. The more you move your body, the more muscle density you create, the better your body gets at it, the better your metabolism becomes, the faster your recovery will be, and the more robust your health will be in the future.

That can mean making sure you get out for nice long walks. Park in the far end of the parking lot. Avoid the elevator and the escalators and take the stairs. Building movement into your day will make your recovery faster and lock in more robust health.

Another important contributor to speeding your recovery is reducing your stress. Chronic stress generates a steady flow of adrenaline and cortisol that has an aging effect, prevents healing, and—critically for our purposes—communicates to your cells that life is unsafe. As long as life is unsafe, the body will be incredibly reluctant to release stored fat. Your psychology, in other words, can play an incredibly important role in helping your body feel comfortable in returning to proper sugar regulation, proper fat storage, and other functions.

Don't take this journey by yourself. There is a saying, variously attributed to different wise elders, that "if you want to go fast, go alone, but if you want to go far, go together." Studies of primates have shown that when they groom each other, that act reduces the stress hormones in both animals. Cortisol and adrenaline levels go down. Those animals that are not groomed by other animals—the lowest in social ranking—do not enjoy that reduction in stress chemicals and, correspondingly, have the shortest lifespans in a group. Spend time strengthening your social connections. We are social animals. When we are denied strong social connections, our bodies produce stress hormones. Taking time to be with people who care about you, and who you care about, will help you on your journey.

Whenever we want to make a shift in our life, when we want to learn a new skill or change a habit, the beginning is always the most difficult part. You have done that. Now, move forward.

Are there things you can get excited about in the next phase? Absolutely, beginning with learning from others. Remember the story about the monkeys who followed the other monkeys in their new home so they learned what to do and what to eat? Find other people who eat like you and who can inspire you to stay on track in the same way—people you can learn from.

We've shared a number of resources throughout the book. Take advantage of them. Take the survey we described in Week 9; we want to learn about your successes and about your failures, so we can build on the successes and find ways to ameliorate the failures.

We would love simply to hear your stories; you may contact us at stories@postdiabetes.com.

Finally, we want to remind you of something we asked you to do at the beginning of this book. We asked you to imagine teaching what you learned to someone. We want you to do that because we know if you did, you would learn more effectively. Yet we had another motive. We hope by this point you are truly energized by the following:

- the enormous changes you have seen in your own health

- the realization that you can live a postdiabetic life

- the knowledge you've gained about yourself, your relationship with food, and the way you've been manipulated by food and drug companies

- the recognition that you can change not only yourself, but the world around you

We invite you to take that energy and channel it. Share what you have learned. This is how change happens: one person, one conversation, one small victory at a time. The diabetes epidemic is a national disaster. It is also millions of quiet personal crises. Your diabetes is not your fault. It was done to you. But you can do something about it. You already *have* done something about it by reading this book and doing the hard work we asked of you.

Don't stop here. Reach out to someone you know. Help them, as you have helped yourself. You can change the world.

Endnotes

Introduction

1. "New CDC Report: More Than 100 Million Americans Have Prediabetes,"
   Centers for Disease Control and Prevention, accessed October 21, 2023,
   https://www.cdc.gov/media/releases/2017/p0718-diabetes-report.html.

Chapter 1

1. Alexandra Sifferlin, "How the Sugar Lobby Skewed Health Research," *Time*,
   September 12, 2016, https://time.com/4485710/sugar-industry-heart
   -disease-research.

2. Ibid.

3. Margot Sanger-Katz, "The Decline of 'Big Soda,'" *The New York Times*,
   October 2, 2015, https://www.nytimes.com/2015/10/04/upshot/soda-
   industry-struggles-as-consumer-tastes-change.html.

4. Anahad O'Connor, "Coca-Cola Funds Scientists Who Shift Blame for Obesity
   Away from Bad Diets," *Well* Blog, March 15, 2016, https://well.blogs.nytimes.
   com/2015/08/09/coca-cola-funds-scientists-who-shift-blame-for-obesity
   -away-from-bad-diets/.

5. Mitchell Glasson and Nolan Lehman, "What's New with Fast-Food Drive-
   Thrus?," *QSR Magazine*, August 29, 2022, https://www.qsrmagazine.com
   /outside-insights/whats-new-fast-food-drive-thrus.

Chapter 2

1. Luise Light, "A Fatally Flawed Food Guide," *Conscious Choice*, last modified
   November 2004, http://web.archive.org/web/20090207074229/http://
   consciouschoice.com/2004/cc1711/wh_lead1711.html.

2. Andrew Dannenberg, Howard Frumkin, and Richard Jackson, *Making
   Healthy Places: Designing and Building for Health, Well-Being, and Sustainability*,
   Amazon, Illustrated edition (Washington, DC: Island Press, 2011).

3. Craig M. Hales et al., "Prevalence of Obesity and Severe Obesity Among
   Adults: United States, 2017–2018," NCHS Data Brief No. 360, February 27,
   2020, https://www.cdc.gov/nchs/products/databriefs/db360.htm.

4. "FastStats—Diabetes," Centers for Disease Control and Prevention, 2019,
   https://www.cdc.gov/nchs/fastats/diabetes.htm.

5. Tim Stickings, "99% of Patients Killed by Coronavirus in Italy Had Existing Illnesses," *Daily Mail*, March 19, 2020, https://www.dailymail.co.uk/news /article-8130479/99-patients-killed-coronavirus-Italy-existing-illnesses-study -finds.html.

6. Roni Caryn Rabin, "Nearly All Patients Hospitalized with Covid-19 Had Chronic Health Issues, Study Finds," *The New York Times*, April 23, 2020, https://www.nytimes.com/2020/04/23/health/coronavirus-patients-risk .html.

7. Edouard Mathieu et al., "Mortality Risk of COVID-19," *Our World in Data*, https://ourworldindata.org/coronavirus.

8. Arthur, "Historical Consumption of Sugar: A Concise Exploration of Its Evolution," Sugar and Sweetener Guide, July 26, 2023, https://www.sugar-and-sweetener-guide.com/historical-consumption-of-sugar/.

9. Nigel Hawkes, "More Doctors Are Disclosing Payments from Drug Companies," *Britih Medical Journal* 357, no. j3195 (June 2017), https://doi .org/10.1136/bmj.j3195.

10. Eric Sagara et al., "Dollars for Docs," ProPublica, last modified September 29, 2014, https://projects.propublica.org/d4d-archive/.

11. Paul Chrystal, *Bioterrorism and Biological Warfare: Disease as a Weapon of War* (South Yorkshire, UK: Pen & Sword Military, 2023).

12. Ellen Daniel, "US Pharma Lobbying Spend Surged to $25.4M in 2017," *Pharmaceutical Technology*, January 26, 2018, https://www.pharmaceutical-technology.com/news/us-pharma-lobbying-spend-surged-25-4m-2017/.

13. "The Cost of Diabetes," American Diabetes Association, 2018, https://www .diabetes.org/resources/statistics/cost-diabetes.

14. Jonathan Chadwick, "Eating Just One Egg a Day Increases Your Risk of Diabetes by 60 Percent, Study Warns," *Daily Mail*, November 16, 2020, https://www.dailymail.co.uk/sciencetech/article-8954561/One-egg-day-increases-risk-developing-diabetes-60-study-warns.html.

15. Mia De Graaf, "One Egg a Day 'LOWERS Your Risk of Type 2 Diabetes': Controversial Study Says It Promotes Fatty Acids That Protect You from the Disease," *Daily Mail*, January 3, 2019, https://www.dailymail.co.uk/health /article-6555491/One-egg-day-LOWERS-risk-type-2-diabetes.html.

Chapter 5

1. "White Lies? Five Milk Myths Debunked," Physicians Committee for Responsible Medicine, February 11, 2016, https://www.pcrm.org/news/blog /white-lies-five-myths-debunked.

Chapter 7

1. "Food, n.," in *Oxford English Dictionary*, n.d., https://www.oed.com /dictionary/food_n?tab=meaning_and_use#3958707.

2. Maria Antonietta Zoroddu et al., "The Essential Metals for Humans: A Brief Overview," *Journal of Inorganic Biochemistry* 195 (June 2019): 120–29, https:// doi.org/10.1016/j.jinorgbio.2019.03.013.

About the Authors

Rubén Ruiz, M.D., is the medical director of three clinics in Los Angeles serving primarily low-income Hispanic residents. He opened his first clinic in 2002. Prior to that, he served patients in similar clinics in Los Angeles, a practice he began soon after graduating from the UCLA School of Medicine in 1982. He completed his own journey into a postdiabetic life in 2018. In the process he dropped 56 pounds. Before then he had taken 10 medications for diabetes, hypertension, cholesterol, thyroid, sinuses, heartburn and insomnia. After he found his new normal, he was down to a single medication for hypertension, saving $12,000 a year in prescription costs.

Eric Edmeades was born in South Africa and raised in Canada. He is an entrepreneur with a varied business history, including mobile computing, Hollywood special effects, military research and development, and the development of award-winning and life-saving medical simulation equipment for the U.S. Army.

In 2011, Eric combined two of his passions—nutritional anthropology and behavioral change dynamics—to create WILDFIT®, the highly effective health transformation coaching company that has now served over 50,000 clients in 130 countries.

For that program, Eric has received the award for the highest-rated program on the Mindvalley platform for two years in a row.

In 2018, Eric was awarded the Senate 150 Medal by the Canadian Senate for his work in empowering people to improve the quality of their lives.

Eric enjoys kiteboarding, wildlife photography, public speaking, and spending time with his two children, Daniel and Zoe.

Acknowledgments

I, Eric, love writing, but finishing books is, well, not my favorite part of the project, and so, with that, I would like to acknowledge both Tucker Max and Scribe Media for their support in birthing this book and getting it out to the world.

I would also like to acknowledge my father, Baz Edmeades, for feeding my curiosity about human history and evolution all these years; many of the thoughts and ideas that have found their way into this book owe their existence to our long verbal expeditions to ancient Africa and a few of our physical ones too.

Further, without the support of the teams at both Mindvalley and WILDFIT, we could never have reached so many people with our message, and I am grateful for their dedication and stalwart support.

Senator Mobina Jaffer is an incredible woman worthy of an entire book of her own, but her interest in my work and the light she has shone upon our results has been a genuine gift and restored (some of) my faith in government. ;-)

J.J. Virgin is a living example of "a rising tide raises all ships," and her encouragement, support, and introductions have been invaluable to me.

I would also like to mention a number of other people who either started me on this road or helped me find my way along it when the lights faded at times. Roughly in order of when they crossed my path, I would like to thank my third grade teacher, Jan Kulchinski; my good friend Tim Ames; Tony Robbins; Cathy Lee Crosby; Simon Reilly; Gavin Wilding; Don Johanson; Gasper Mbise; and Nnona, a Hadza chief.

Lastly, I would like to acknowledge some forward-thinking doctors that are doing excellent work in metabolic health, including Dr. Loren Cordain, Dr. Aseem Malhotra, Dr. Tro Kalayjian, Dr. Neelima Deshpande, and Professor Tim Noakes.

While Rubén and I have had many influences in the development of this book, any errors, omissions, or assumptions are entirely ours.

Appendix

WILDFIT Spring Recipes

BREAKFAST

Bacon-Avocado-Ranch Egg Muffins
Time: 45 minutes
Serves: 6

Ranch Seasoning Mix

2 teaspoons chives

3 teaspoons dried dill weed

4 teaspoons garlic powder

4 teaspoons onion powder

4 tablespoons parsley

2 teaspoons black pepper

1 teaspoon sea salt

Muffin Ingredients

Drizzle of olive oil

2 large avocados, diced

6 strips of bacon, cooked crispy
(free from nitrates, sugar, and
additives)

12 whole eggs, whisked (or 3 cups
egg whites only)

Preparation
Preheat the oven to 350°F.

In a small bowl thoroughly mix the ranch seasoning.

Grease a 12-cup muffin tin generously with olive oil.

Divide the diced avocado into the 12 muffin cups.

Crumble the bacon into pieces and put about ½ a slice of crumbles on top of the avocado in each cup, then sprinkle ¼ teaspoon of ranch seasoning over the top of each one.

Whisk the eggs with the remaining ranch seasoning, then divide the egg mixture into each cup. Each cup should be almost full.

Bake for 22 to 30 minutes or until the eggs are baked through.

Baked Eggs in Portobello Mushroom Caps

Time: 45 minutes
Serves: 6

Ingredients

6 portobello mushroom caps

Drizzle of olive oil

12 prosciutto slices

6 farm fresh eggs

Ground black pepper, to taste

Fresh parsley or thyme

Preparation

Preheat the oven to 375°F.

Carefully clean the portobello mushroom caps with a damp cloth. Remove the stem and scrape out insides to create a well to fit the egg.

Rub a little olive oil on the outside of the mushrooms. This will keep them from sticking to the pan.

Arrange the mushroom caps on a 9 x 12-inch baking sheet.

Place 1 or 2 slices of prosciutto inside each mushroom cap.

Carefully pour an egg onto a prosciutto-filled mushroom cap.

Sprinkle with black pepper and fresh herbs of choice. Salt is not recommended since the prosciutto is already salty.

Place the baking pan into the oven.

Bake for 20 to 30 minutes. The amount of cook time required varies depending on how thick your mushrooms are and how cooked you like your eggs.

Crustless Quiche

Time: 45 minutes
Serves: 4 to 5

Ingredients

4 to 6 pieces of pork sausage or bacon (without nitrates, sugar, or additives)

2 cups of chopped greens (spinach, kale, or finely chopped broccoli)

12 eggs

Sea salt (optional)

Liberal amount of ground pepper

1 teaspoon coconut oil (used on the pan)

Preparation

Preheat the oven to 350°F.

Chop the sausage into pieces and partially cook it in a skillet.

Add the greens and soften them. You can put a lid on to speed up this process.

Whisk the eggs in a bowl with salt and pepper.

Grease a 9-inch pie pan with the coconut oil. Pour the blended eggs into the pan.

Add the veggie and meat mixture to the top of the eggs. Doing it this way keeps them from all sinking to the bottom middle of the pan when you pour.

Bake for 30 to 35 minutes.

Let the quiche cool before cutting it into 4 or 5 pieces. Put the pieces into individual containers for 4 or 5 mornings' worth of easy breakfasts!

Easy Egg Wraps

Time: 5 minutes
Serves: 1

Ingredients

Drizzle of avocado oil

1 egg

Optional seasonings: salt, pepper, paprika, cayenne pepper, basil, oregano, etc.

Optional fillings: turkey, avocado, and bacon

Preparation

Heat a small skillet over medium heat. Grease it with avocado oil.

In a bowl, crack the egg and mix well with a fork.

Pour the egg into the hot pan and tilt the pan to spread it into a large circle on the bottom of the pan.

Let it cook 30 seconds. (Sprinkle with seasonings if desired.)

Carefully flip the egg with a large spatula and let it cook another 30 seconds.

Remove the egg wrap from pan.

Let the egg wrap cool slightly (or fully), top as desired with fillings, roll, and serve warm or cold.

SMOOTHIES

Alkagizer Prime

Time: 5 minutes
Serves: 2

Ingredients

5 stalks celery, chopped

5 inches cucumber, chopped

1 avocado, chopped

2 handfuls spinach, chopped

1 handful collard greens, chopped

1 handful kale, chopped

Juice of 1 lemon

1 handful cilantro

½ inch fresh jalapeño pepper
(adjust to taste)

Preparation

Add the celery, cucumber, avocado, spinach, greens, and kale to the blender. Add the lemon juice, cilantro, and jalapeño pepper. Blend.

Pour over ice and drink immediately. Can be stored in an airtight container such as a mason jar for up to 3 days.

SALADS

Avocado Chicken Salad Wraps

Time: 5 minutes
Serves: 8

Ingredients

1 ripe avocado, peeled and pitted

1 tablespoon lime juice*

2 tablespoons minced fresh cilantro

2 tablespoons minced red onion

½ teaspoon garlic powder

2 cooked boneless, skinless chicken breasts, cut into ½-inch cubes (about 2 cups)

Salt and pepper to taste

8 to 10 butter lettuce leaves

Preparation

In a medium bowl, mash the avocado with the lime juice. Stir in the cilantro, onion, garlic powder, and chicken cubes until just combined. Season the chicken salad with salt and pepper to taste.

Just before serving, fill the butter lettuce leaves with chicken salad and serve immediately.

---

* Use only a few drops in WILDFIT Spring.

Spinach Salad with Creamy Avocado Dressing
Time: 5 minutes
Serves: 8

Spinach Salad Ingredients

4 cups washed spinach leaves, torn into bite-sized pieces

4 strips bacon, cooked until crispy (free from nitrates, sugar, and additives)

2 eggs, hard-boiled and peeled

6 to 8 Cremini mushrooms, sliced thinly

¼ cup red onion, sliced thinly

Dairy-Free Avocado Cream

1 cup loosely packed cilantro

½ large avocado

Juice of ½ lime†

1 clove garlic

¼ cup olive oil

½ tablespoon apple cider vinegar or white wine vinegar‡

Pinch of sea salt

Preparation

Arrange the salad items in a large bowl.

Blend the avocado cream ingredients together in a food processor.

Drizzle the avocado cream on the salad and serve.

---

† Use only a couple of drops in WILDFIT Spring.

‡ Omit or use only a couple of drops in WILDFIT Spring.

SOUPS

Bone Broth

Time: 10 minutes to prep, 6 hours to cook
Serves: 8

Ingredients

Grass-fed beef bones, chicken carcass, or any mixture of bones from wild or pasture-raised, healthy animals

12 to 16 cups purified water

Salt and pepper to taste

Preparation

Place the bones into a large slow cooker. Only a few are needed; however, the more you can fit into the cooker, the more nutritious the broth will be.

Fill the cooker with enough filtered water to cover the bones, leaving about three inches at the top of the pot.

Set the cooker on low and cook for a minimum of 6 hours. Poultry bones can cook for up to 24 hours and beef bones can simmer for up to 48 hours.

Allow the cooker to cool and pour the broth through a sieve into a storage container, or use tongs to remove all bones.

Season with salt and pepper to taste.

Enjoy this nutrient-dense broth within 5 to 7 days or freeze for later. Tip: Freeze broth in ice cube trays for added convenience.

Creamy Cauliflower Soup

Time: 35 minutes
Serves: 8

Ingredients

½ tablespoon olive oil

1 onion, diced

2 cloves garlic, minced

1 head cauliflower, diced

32 ounces vegetable broth

1 teaspoon salt

Sliced green onions for serving, if desired

Preparation

In a heavy pot, heat the olive oil on medium heat.

Add the onion and garlic. Cook until soft, approximately 5 minutes.

Add the cauliflower and vegetable broth.

Bring the mixture to a boil, then cover and simmer until the cauliflower softens, approximately 15 to 20 minutes.

Pour the contents into a blender, add salt to taste, and blend until smooth.

Note: You can make this in a slow cooker. Add all the ingredients and cook on low for 3 to 5 hours. The flavor is the same, but the consistency won't be as thick. To troubleshoot that, you can remove the slow cooker lid for the last hour of cooking so some of the liquid evaporates.

Creamy Leek Soup

Time: 10 minutes prep time, 20 minutes cook time
Serves: 4 to 6

Ingredients

2 large leeks, washed well, dark green ends removed, roughly chopped (about 3 cups)

1 medium cauliflower, cored and roughly chopped (4 to 5 cups)

1 medium onion, diced (about 1 cup)

4 cups chicken broth

1 cup coconut milk

Salt and pepper to taste

Preparation

Add the leeks, cauliflower, onion, chicken broth, and coconut milk to a large soup pot.

Bring the mixture to a boil, then reduce to a simmer for about 20 minutes or until all the veggies are tender.

Allow the soup to cool, then puree it until smooth using a blender. Be careful: You may need to do 2 or more batches so the blender doesn't overflow.

Season with salt and pepper to taste.

Note: You can make this in a slow cooker. Add all the ingredients and cook on low for 3 to 5 hours. The flavor is the same, but the consistency won't be as thick. To troubleshoot that, you can remove the slow cooker lid for the last hour of cooking so some of the liquids evaporate.

SNACKS

Cucumber Wraps

Time: 5 minutes
Serves: 1

Ingredients

¼ of a cucumber, peeled and
   sliced thinly lengthwise

3 slices unprocessed turkey

Half a tomato, diced*

¼ of a carrot, shredded†

3 leaves of lettuce, shredded

Preparation

Lay 4 cucumber slices on a cutting board lengthwise next to each other so the edges slightly overlap.

Layer the thinly sliced turkey on top of the sliced cucumbers.

Add the sliced veggies on top of the turkey in a line to the side.

Roll tightly into a nice wrap.

Use a paring or serrated knife and slice between each cucumber slice. Enjoy!

---

*   Omit for WILDFIT Spring.

†   Omit for WILDFIT Spring.

Kale Chips

Time: 5 minutes prep, 20 minutes cook time
Serves: 4

Ingredients

1 head of kale, washed and dried completely

2 tablespoons olive oil
1 teaspoon sea salt

Preparation

Preheat the oven to 275°F.

Remove the ribs from the kale and cut into 1½-inch pieces.

Place the kale pieces on a 15 x 21-inch baking sheet and toss with the olive oil and salt.

Bake the kale pieces until they are crisp, turning the leaves halfway through, about 20 minutes.

Zucchini Chips

Time: 25 minutes prep, 2½ hours cook time
Serves: 4

Ingredients

2 zucchini, well washed and sliced

2 teaspoons olive or coconut oil, divided
Salt and pepper, to taste

Preparation

Preheat the oven to 230°F.

Slice the zucchini on a mandoline into ⅛-inch-thick chips.

Lay the zucchini chips out on a paper towel. Let them sit for 20 minutes.

Pat dry any excess moisture from the zucchini.

In a large bowl, lightly toss them with 1 teaspoon of olive oil and the salt and pepper.

Prep a 15 x 21-inch baking sheet with the remaining 1 teaspoon oil.

Bake 2½ hours, or until crisp.

ENTREES

Almond-Crusted Chicken with Lemon Zucchini Noodles

Time: 10 minutes prep time, 15 minutes cook time
Serves: 2

Ingredients

⅓ cup almonds

1 egg

1 (10-ounce) chicken breast

1 tablespoon extra-virgin olive oil

2 medium zucchini

2 carrots‡

1 fresh lemon

¼ teaspoon garlic salt

Pepper to taste

Preparation

In a high-speed food processor, process the almonds until you have a powder.

Add the almonds to a plate. Break the egg onto a second plate, and whisk it.

Cut the chicken breast in half by slicing it lengthwise. Using a tenderizer, pound out both sides of each half.

Take one chicken breast half and coat it completely in the egg. Then, coat each side of the chicken half in the almonds. Repeat with the other chicken breast half.

Heat the olive oil in a large skillet over medium heat. Make sure the oil coats the bottom of the skillet. Then add both chicken breast halves. Cook for 5 minutes on one side, then flip.

While the chicken is cooking, chop or spiralize the zucchini and carrots.

Slice the lemon in half. Cut one half into thin slices.

Once the chicken is done, set it aside on a plate. Add the vegetables to the skillet.

Squeeze the remaining lemon wedge over the vegetables and add the garlic salt and pepper. Stir the vegetables until they are slightly cooked down, about 2 minutes. Move the vegetable noodles to one side of the

‡   Omit for WILDFIT Spring or substitute zucchini.

skillet and lightly brown the lemon slices on both sides, about 1 minute each side.

Dress the plates with vegetable noodles, then add the almond-crusted chicken. Garnish with lemon slices.

Avocado and Bacon Zoodles

Time: 15 minutes
Serves: 4

Ingredients

1 ripe California avocado

1 jalapeño, chopped, seeds removed

1 clove garlic

2 tablespoons freshly squeezed lime juice

2 tablespoons chopped fresh cilantro

1 tablespoon avocado oil

⅛ to ¼ teaspoon chipotle powder or chili powder

Salt and pepper to taste

4 medium zucchini, spiralized

4 slices bacon, cooked crisp and crumbled (free from nitrates, sugar, and additives)

Preparation

In a blender or food processor, combine the avocado, jalapeño, garlic, lime juice, cilantro, avocado oil, chipotle powder, and salt and pepper. Blend until smooth. Add 2 to 4 tablespoons of water and continue to process until a thick but pourable consistency is achieved.

Cook the zucchini uncovered in the microwave for 1 or 2 minutes on high, until hot and just tender.

Divide the spiralized zucchini among 4 plates and top with the avocado sauce and crumbled bacon. Serve warm.

Baked Salmon Pouches

Time: 5 minutes prep time, 20 minutes cook time
Serves: 2

Ingredients

2 medium zucchini, halved
   lengthwise and thinly sliced
¼ red onion, thinly sliced
1 teaspoon fresh dill, chopped
2 slices lemon

Drizzle of extra-virgin olive oil
Salt and freshly ground pepper
Two 6-ounce salmon fillets
Few drops of fresh lemon juice

Preparation

Preheat the oven to 350°F.

Prepare 2 large pieces of parchment paper by folding them in half to crease. Then open the papers and lay them flat.

On one side of the crease, place half of the zucchini, the red onion, the dill, and one lemon slice. Drizzle with the olive oil and sprinkle with salt and pepper.

Place a salmon fillet on top and drizzle with the lemon juice. Season with salt and pepper. Repeat with the second piece of parchment paper and remaining ingredients.

Fold the parchment paper over the salmon to close, making a half-moon shape. Seal the open sides by folding small pleats in the paper.

Place the parchment packets on a 15 x 21-inch rimmed baking sheet and bake for 15 to 20 minutes until the salmon is opaque. Serve warm.

Chili Beef Lettuce Wraps

Time: 5 minutes prep, 15 minutes cooking
Serves: 3 to 4

Ingredients

2 teaspoons neutral-flavored oil, like coconut, avocado, or walnut

1 pound lean ground beef

1 tablespoon fish sauce

1 to 2 tablespoons chili sauce (depending on how much heat you want)

2 tablespoons filtered water

1 large lime, zested and juiced (about 1½ tablespoons juice)§

¼ cup thinly sliced green onions

½ cup chopped cilantro

1 to 2 heads iceberg lettuce, washed and cut into cups

Preparation

Heat the oil in a large frying pan over medium-high heat, then cook the beef until it's cooked through and starting to brown, breaking it apart with a spatula as it cooks.

While the beef cooks, mix together the fish sauce, chili sauce, and water in a small bowl. Add the lime juice and lime zest.

When the beef is done, add the chili sauce mixture to the pan and let it sizzle until the water has evaporated, stirring a few times to get the flavor mixed through the meat. Turn off the heat and stir in the lime zest, lime juice, sliced green onions, and chopped cilantro.

Put the meat mixture in the iceberg lettuce leaves and wrap the lettuce around it.

§   Omit for WILDFIT Spring.

Garlic Bacon Avocado Burgers

Time: 15 minutes
Serves: 7

Ingredients

½ pound bacon (free from
   nitrates, sugar, and additives)

6 large cloves garlic

1¼ pounds ground beef

¼ teaspoon pink Himalayan
   sea salt

¼ teaspoon fresh cracked pepper

1 avocado

Preparation

Using a food processor, pulse the bacon strips until they are ground.

Crush or mince the garlic and place it in a large bowl. Add the ground beef and bacon into the bowl. Sprinkle the salt and pepper over the meat. Using your hands, combine the meats, garlic, and seasoning until well mixed.

Divide the meat into ¼-pound sections and shape into round, flat patties.

Heat a large cast iron skillet (or a frying pan) over medium or high heat. Once the skillet is heated, add the patties in batches and sear for about 3 to 4 minutes per side.

Serve with a few avocado slices on top of each burger.

Garlic Shrimp

Time: 5 minutes prep time, 10 minutes cook time
Serves: 4

Ingredients

¼ cup extra-virgin olive oil

10 garlic cloves, thinly sliced

1 pound large or jumbo shrimp, peeled and deveined, tails removed if desired

¾ teaspoon sea salt

¼ teaspoon freshly ground pepper

¼ teaspoon smoked paprika

Pinch of cayenne pepper

Preparation

Heat the olive oil in a large heavy skillet over medium-low heat. Add the garlic and cook, stirring frequently, until it is softened but not browned, about 5 minutes.

Add the shrimp in a single layer, raise the heat to medium-high, and sprinkle on the salt, pepper, paprika, and cayenne.

Cook the shrimp until it turns pink on the bottom, 2 to 3 minutes.

Flip and cook until the shrimp are opaque throughout, another 2 to 3 minutes. Serve hot.

SIDES

Cauliflower Rice

Time: 5 minutes prep, 5 to 8 minutes cook time
Serves: 4

Ingredients

1 large head of cauliflower,
 washed and thoroughly dried
 and cut into 4 even sections

1 tablespoon olive oil
Salt and pepper to taste

Preparation

Use a box grater with medium-sized holes or a food processor with the grater attachment to grate the cauliflower into the size of rice, leaving any large, tough stems behind.

Transfer the riced cauliflower to a clean towel or paper towel and press to remove any excess moisture, which can make your dish soggy.

Once you have your cauliflower rice, it's easy to cook! Simply sauté it in a large skillet over medium heat in olive oil. Cover with a lid so the cauliflower steams and becomes more tender. Cook for 5 to 8 minutes, then season as desired (such as with soy sauce¶ or salt and pepper).

¶   Soy sauce is not WILDFIT approved.

Sauteed Broccoli Rabe with Garlic & Oil

Time: 5 minutes prep, 5 minutes cook time
Serves: 4

Ingredients

2 teaspoons kosher salt, divided

1 bunch broccoli rabe (about 16 ounces), stems trimmed and cut into 2-inch pieces

1 tablespoon olive oil

5 garlic cloves, thinly sliced

¼ teaspoon crushed red pepper flakes

Preparation

Bring a large pot of water with 4 liters of water and 1 teaspoon of salt to a boil.

Add the broccoli rabe and cook until slightly tender and bright green, about 2 minutes. Drain and set aside.

Heat a large, deep nonstick sauté pan over medium-high heat.

Add the olive oil and garlic and cook, stirring frequently, until the garlic is golden, for about 1 minute.

Add the broccoli rabe, pepper flakes, and the remaining 1 teaspoon salt. Keep stirring until heated through, 2 to 3 minutes. Serve hot!

Index

Z

Notes

Notes

Notes

_____

_____

_____

_____

_____

_____

_____

_____

_____

_____

_____

_____

_____

_____

_____

Notes

———————————————————————————

———————————————————————————

———————————————————————————

———————————————————————————

———————————————————————————

———————————————————————————

———————————————————————————

———————————————————————————

———————————————————————————

———————————————————————————

———————————————————————————

———————————————————————————

———————————————————————————

———————————————————————————

———————————————————————————

———————————————————————————

———————————————————————————

———————————————————————————

Hay House Titles of Related Interest

YOU CAN HEAL YOUR LIFE, the movie,
starring Louise Hay & Friends
(available as an online streaming video)
www.hayhouse.com/louise-movie

THE SHIFT, the movie,
starring Dr. Wayne W. Dyer
(available as an online streaming video)
www.hayhouse.com/the-shift-movie

***

*GROW A NEW BODY: How Spirit and Power Plant Nutrients
Can Transform Your Health,* by Dr. Alberto Villoldo

*HEALTHY AT LAST: A Plant-Based Approach to Preventing
and Reversing Diabetes and Other Chronic Illnesses,* by Eric Adams

*FOOD BABE KITCHEN: More than 100 Delicious, Real Food Recipes
to Change Your Body and Your Life,* by Vani Hari

REAL SUPERFOODS: Everyday Ingredients to Elevate Your Health,
by Ocean Robbins and Nichole Dandrea-Russert, MS, RDN

All of the above are available at your local bookstore,
or may be ordered by contacting Hay House (see next page).

***

We hope you enjoyed this Hay House book. If you'd like to receive our online catalog featuring additional information on Hay House books and products, or if you'd like to find out more about the Hay Foundation, please contact:

Hay House LLC, P.O. Box 5100, Carlsbad, CA 92018-5100
(760) 431-7695 or (800) 654-5126
www.hayhouse.com® • www.hayfoundation.org

———

Published in Australia by:
Hay House Australia Publishing Pty Ltd
18/36 Ralph St., Alexandria NSW 2015
Phone: +61 (02) 9669 4299
www.hayhouse.com.au

Published in the United Kingdom by:
Hay House UK Ltd
1st Floor, Crawford Corner,
91–93 Baker Street, London W1U 6QQ
Phone: +44 (0)20 3927 7290
www.hayhouse.co.uk

Published in India by:
Hay House Publishers (India) Pvt Ltd
Muskaan Complex, Plot No. 3,
B-2, Vasant Kunj, New Delhi 110 070
Phone: +91 11 41761620
www.hayhouse.co.in

———

Let Your Soul Grow

Experience life-changing transformation—one video
at a time—with guidance from the world's leading experts.

www.healyourlifeplus.com

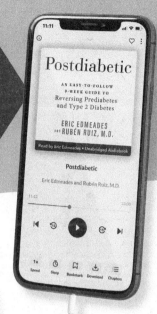